Occupy Your Body:

The Personal Wellness Revolution

Kimberly Ciano

Occupy Your Body:
The Personal Wellness Revolution

Copyright @ 2015 by Kimberly Ciano

Use this for health related content:
The content of this book is for general instruction only. Each person's physical, emotional, and spiritual condition is unique. The instruction in this book is not intended to replace or interrupt the reader's relationship with a physician or other professional. Please consult your doctor for matters pertaining to your specific health and diet.

To contact the publisher, visit www.createspace.com
To contact the author, visit www.unearthyourwarrior.com

978-0-692-57981-7

Printed in the United States of America

Flow of Content

Namasté

I honor the place in you in which the entire Universe dwells
The place of Love, of Truth, of Light & of Peace
When you are in that place in you and I am in that place in me
We Are One.

There are many people without whom this book would not have become a reality. I would like to thank my parents for being such critical sources of strength in my life. Without your encouragement and support, I may not have found the courage to publish this book and share this information with the world.

I must express the deepest gratitude to YOU, my readers! Whether you have been a supporting friend or we are complete strangers, you are my inspiration. This book is for you and I sincerely hope that you find within these pages the tools you need to occupy your body, live your truth authentically, and to discover the happiness that is held within.

A special thanks goes to the very talented friends who contributed their talents to make this book come to life:

Joshua Paull Photography
jpaullphoto@gmail.com

Matthew Grotta
Cover Design
matthewgrotta@live.com

Devin Grotta
Professional Hairstylist & Makeup Artist
devingrotta@gmail.com

Hannah M. Hicks
Editorial Assistant, Public Integrity
Hhicks1@pride.hofstra.edu

Dedication

This book is dedicated to Joshua Rosenthal and the Institute for Integrative Nutrition™. Without the guidance and support that I have received, even after graduating from IIN, this book would not have become a reality.

Thank you for sharing the knowledge that empowered me to find authentic wellness, occupy my body, and work towards building the life of health and happiness that I now know I deserve.

Introduction

To better acquaint you, my wonderful reader with the Occupy Your Body movement, we will start at the beginning. You found this book, or more-so were found by this book, because you feel a desire for growth and for change. There is something in your life that is making you ill or is holding you back from finding the delicate flow of optimal health and wellness. The good news is that you are not alone and the better news is that you have the capacity to grow. I would like to invite you to begin with an exercise that will be very brief and will require your full attention.

Turn off the television or the background noise and get comfortable in a seated position. Create length in the spine by grounding down into the sit-bones and lifting up through the crown of your head. Find a deep restorative inhale and release a long and calming exhale.

Now, imagine what it is in your life that you desire to change; allow yourself to observe the physical reaction of your body and the feelings attached to these thoughts while they enter your mind.

How do you feel?
How do you envision your life a day, a month, and a year from now if you do not find change?
How will living with this pain impact your health and happiness in the future?
What are the emotions associated with the idea of continuing without change?

Maintain a deep and fulfilling breath, inhaling through the diaphragm and exhaling with intention. Now, imagine what your life would be like if you found a way to overcome this pain, to evolve beyond the limitations imposed by what is keeping you in pain. Close your eyes for a moment and allow the vision of a life of growth and wellness to flourish in your mind.

How does this vision of wellness make you feel?
Did you notice any changes in how your body
reacted to each scenario?
What was it about your life that changed?
What are the emotions associated with the vision
of living a life of wellness?

It is important to remind ourselves each and every day that we are in the driver's seat on this journey towards finding a flow of health and happiness. To do this we must observe our feelings, both physical and emotional, to better understand not only what it is we want but why we want it. This idea of asserting a "Why" is a powerful motivator for staying on track when faced with the task of building life changes that will endure and last. Visualization is a powerful tool to transform what we imagine within our mind into something we experience in our perceived reality.

In the following sections of the book, practice opening your eyes and allow yourself to fully interact with the valuable information being shared. The life of wellness you just envisioned is waiting for you to wake up and live it.

∞

In contrast to the division of ideas that couples with chapter books, the content within this book flows fluidly to correlate with the many concepts within it. It is important to reconstruct our scope of understanding and view the ideas being presented from a holistic perspective. In order to reflect on the important information being presented, read each part with a critical lens and pause briefly before moving on. Each section begins by presenting the aspect of wellness that will be addressed: achieving physical health, living presently in the moment, and thriving through conscious thought. Within each section, subsections will follow that present comparisons and ideas to further explore each aspect of wellness. The section will then end with the introduction of practical tips and tools, such as exercises and meditations, which are to be utilized and built into your daily routine and lifestyle.

While reading, keep in mind to enjoy the process. Happiness and wellness are not destinations; they are continual journeys that can only be found through action and consistency. View this book as an instrument to help you begin navigating your path. At the end, once you begin to implement the information and exercises into your life, you will have the bearings to sail forward and actively participate in your journey for wellness!

You are a conscious being with a miraculous body that always strives for balance and health and you are capable of choosing a life that supports authentic wellness and exponential happiness.

"Happiness depends on ourselves."
-Aristotle

Kimberly and the Case of the Mysterious Heart Ache

Living like My Body was on Loan

Holding the frame in my hands, I searched for that feeling of pride that had been promised to me.

Nothing

I could feel nothing, with the exception of that familiar burn from the vodka in my empty stomach. Taking another sip, my whole body seemed to warm from the inside out. My fingers traced the edge of the frame I had purchased on sale at the arts and crafts store. I could see my face reflected in the glass that was protecting my precious college degree from any wear or tear. My eyes were dull, glaring back at me through the warped reflection as the seal of the university shimmered in gold and my full name stared back at me, boldly printed across the paper.

This was it: the climax and the empty aftermath of all my years of hard work. I had heard once that the French refer to an orgasm as *la petite mort* or "the little death". It refers to the melancholy that follows a climactic build; a loss of life force energy one faces after the ecstasy of sharing oneself with another. Where I should be immersed in the bliss of my accomplishments, I felt empty in optimism. At least my glass of vodka was half full.

I pressed my back against the wall and collapsed under the weight of that weightless piece of paper. Looking around my room, it felt like a strange place. I moved back home with my parents after graduation and had to leave the apartment that I had turned into my own home and shared with friends. This was my childhood house, so why did it feel so foreign. What had changed?

The air in the room smelled like any other Long Island summer and I could hear the soft song of crickets from outside the window. A cool breeze filtered through the screens and danced across my legs. I looked down at my thighs and was suddenly very aware of how thin I had become over the past two years.

When was the last time I ate?

I wasn't sure. I worked long and odd hours. Eating and sleeping were no longer a priority. Making money and self-medicating had called shot gun in the journey of my life. Where was I heading? To freedom, of course. Towards independence and happiness. How I was going to get to that place, I was unsure. I believed I had taken a few wrong turns and the first had been in my decision to attend a private university.

"You are too smart for community college," my guidance counselor had advised me four years before that night, "to be competitive in the corporate world, you must get a degree from a private and prestigious university."

Looking back down at my hands and my degree, my reflection now seemed to mock me. I signed my freedom away to the loan companies to acquire this degree—the piece of paper that was supposed to open all doors to opportunity and freedom. All of the nights spent awake in the library studying for tests and writing papers, the nights spent awake at the bars with friends drinking and laughing, networking and making connections, the person I had become over these past four years, stared back at me. I took another sip of vodka and felt burning; a warmth inside of me deeper than my stomach. A sour spark of bitterness consumed me.

This is not what was promised to me. This is not what I was told.

I had always done what was expected. I prided myself on achieving awards for my academics, on having an extensive resume, on working hard to build a future for myself. A box sat in my closet holding all the little trinkets and certificates that branded me a success throughout the course of my life. I wanted to scream. I wanted to have a fit and tear down everything on the walls in my room.

Was this it? Would I be forced to take any job that made me enough money to pay bills? Could I find my path to freedom while being bound to such a large number in debt?

Rage began to overwhelm the bitterness. My entire body became flushed with a fever of anger and I felt sick to my stomach. My thoughts began to swim drunkenly through my head. I pressed up to my feet and threw the frame across the room. I heard the shatter of glass and then the sound of my heart racing in the silence. After finding the bottom of my drinking glass, I closed my eyes and drifted into a dreamless sleep.

∞

I spent the next year of my life carrying around the anger that I had found that night; wearing my resentment for society like a shield while burning inside with that familiar bitterness. I had begun to punish myself daily because I could not punish the world and circumstances that surrounded me. I continued on with my volatile relationship with alcohol, battled with a nicotine addiction, ate when I absolutely felt the need, and slept for a good portion of my day. Working until three in the morning, I felt as if I could not get anything done for myself without sacrificing sleep.

I battled against my loan company and their demands for monthly payments of sixteen hundred dollars, yet I still paid the cost of a small mortgage each month. All of the money I made that did not go to bills and loans, I began to hoard into savings. New clothes were not necessary until the old fell apart at the seams. My hair only really needed to be cut twice a year, I figured. Whatever food was the cheapest and most convenient would save, not only time, but money.

Had I truly become this defeated?

∞

I was twenty-three years old the night I was at work and felt my limbs go numb. It began as pins-and-needles in my fingers and toes and slowly spread up my arms and legs. An immense weight sunk down on my chest and my lungs felt as if they had sprung a leak. Where was my heartbeat? I had never been aware that my pulse was something I could consciously lose—like car keys or a lighter. I placed two dead, numb fingers on my wrist. Repositioning my fingers in vain, I searched for that familiar beat. Panic set in.

"Are you alright, Kim?" the barback asked me or at least I thought that was what he said.

Stumbling, I made my way out from behind the bar and to the bathroom. Why was it so cold in there? I sat on the toilet and tried to inhale deeply.

You are okay, Kim. Everything will be okay. You're just tired or something. You'll be able to go home soon.

Panic. A surge of adrenaline and I found my heartbeat, except it wasn't the normal rhythmic tune. Instead, a thousand tribal drums exploded from within my ribcage. Pain surged from my chest and began to radiate throughout my body, awakening my dead limbs. The walls of the bathroom began to close and squeeze the life out from within.

Get out of here. You're going to die.

I pressed open the door to the narrow hallway and a ringing began to crescendo in my ears. My vision began to blur as black spots appeared in my path and a dark tunnel started to cave in from my peripheral. The weight that bore down on my knees from my body seemed like an impossible burden and I knew that I was about to lose consciousness. I felt the color drain from my flesh as I approached my boss; paleness crept over my skin like moonlight.

"I...I...my heart, can't breathe," words were forced from my mouth.

Before long, I sat in the back of an ambulance; oxygen mask strapped uncomfortably around my face and questions being asked by the EMT leaning over my stretcher. I had never been in an ambulance before that moment and I came to understand that I never wanted to sit in the back of that fast-moving box again. Trying to inhale slowly to fill my deflating lungs, the ringing in my ears grew louder.

We're here at the hospital? Had I lost consciousness? How much time had passed?

As the intravenous needle pierced a vein in my right arm I could feel the salty burn from the saline meet my bloodstream. Time began to lapse. Tests were done and within a few hours, the ER doctor made his brief guest appearance.

"Well, Miss Ciano, we did tests and could not find anything medically wrong with you," he said. "Your blood test results showed a minor potassium deficiency so I am going to give you a few potassium supplements and we will have you out of here within the hour. Please follow up with your physician tomorrow and if the symptoms persist, come back to the ER."

I could not tell which part of that night had been more distressing—the terrifying symptoms I had suffered, or the fact that there seemed to be no explanation for the phantom illness. With much hesitation, I called my father for a ride and left the hospital feeling slightly worse than when I had arrived.

∞

The next day, I followed up with my physician. Entering his office, I felt faint and weak-hearted. My pulse felt slow and muffled inside my head, like when one lays down in a dark silence and covers their ears with their hands. As I sat in the waiting room, watching reruns of Seinfeld, time slowly came to a stop. My stomach turned inside of my core as if my body was a stalling engine. Being outside of my house was unbearable. At least if my heart gave out, I was in a doctor's office.

"Well Miss Ciano," my physician began with a curt tone, "the ER doctor could not find anything wrong with you and I must say that I do not see anything medically wrong. I am going to recommend you to a cardiologist, but I would suggest seeing a psychiatrist if these symptoms persist. In my opinion, it would appear that your symptoms are psychosomatic."

I felt mocked. I felt as if I had not been taken seriously. These symptoms arrived before the panic had set in. I spent a lot of money studying psychology at a private university, I had wanted to yell but instead, I made an appointment to begin seeing the recommended cardiologist.

Nothing

The cardiologist had found nothing "medically wrong" with me and had no explanation for my persistent symptoms. It had been over a week since I made the initial appointment and over the course of the following week, I had submitted to a series of tests. Those two weeks of my life were a living hell. My bed became a sanctuary—the only place I felt truly safe from my symptoms. If I lost consciousness while lying down, my head would not smack against a floor. If I felt that constant gripping pain in my heart grow worse, I would have someone in my family available to help. Leaving my house was a nightmare; a very real and urgent sense of dread from which I could not escape followed me everywhere I went. At work, I pretended as if nothing were wrong. A fake smile plastered across my face, as real as paper mâché—painted and decorated on the outside, but hollow and empty on the inside. I was becoming a recluse, only leaving my room when it was absolutely necessary.

Emily Dickinson was an agoraphobic and look at all she accomplished.

Placing my hand over my heart I could only feel the endless tingle that had taken up residence in my fingers over the past few weeks. A crushing disappointment sat on top of my chest with a weight that made me feel less alive with every passing moment. I sat across from the cardiologist and closed my eyes. I could not tell if I needed to retch or run away.

∞

"Miss Ciano, fortunately, we could find nothing medically wrong with your heart. I could recommend you to a neurologist but there is nothing further we can do to help you here."

The air outside had changed; the crisp autumn air lost its annual battle against the chill of winter. Sitting in my car, I felt an intense chill inside my bones and my muscles began to tense and twitch. My eyes, however, began to overflow with the hot tears that I held back in the doctor's office. Overwhelmed with frustration, I refused his recommendation to see a neurologist. I was done participating in the game of medical musical chairs in which I had been entered; with every visit, the chair was pulled out from underneath me and I wound up in tears. The only question was what to do next.

"In the long run, we shape our lives, and we shape ourselves. The process never ends until we die. And the choices we make are ultimately our own responsibility."
— Eleanor Roosevelt

How I Chose to Stop Outsourcing My Health

Over the next few weeks, I felt little improvement in my condition and little relief from the symptoms. I woke up feeling hopeless and fell asleep snuggling my apathy and resignation. The days faded together in my memory before I even allowed them the chance to make their mark in time. If the doctors could not help me, I would never be able to help myself. I gave up on my search for a solution. That is, until my boyfriend asked me to see a Holistic doctor.

Looking at the preliminary questionnaire that was e-mailed to me prior to the initial consultation, I was exhausted by its length. The packet was about twenty pages and involved a broad range of questions that were both personal and intensive. An entire medical, psychological and emotional history of my health was required, as well as a summary of my lifestyle habits. I stared blankly at the computer screen as I became overwhelmed by a sudden feeling of shame. Before even writing down my answers to those questions, I was aware of my guilt in the causation of my own suffering. Maybe the culprit of my illness hadn't been some natural defect in the biology of my body but instead there was a flaw in the design of how I had been living my life.

Sitting in the office a week later, my legs bounced with anticipation. I imagined that I would finally have resolution, but I also envisioned a large finger of blame being pointed in my face. The florescent lights and smell of sterility that occupy a doctor's office always caused feelings of unease. I felt exposed under those lights: immaterial and vulnerable.

Please let this nightmare end today, I pleaded repetitively in a silent corner of my mind.

The holistic doctor, Doctor G, addressed me by my first name and spoke to me with an empathy that I had not typically received from any figure of authority. After asking me each question that I had already filled out in the questionnaire in his thick, but soft accent, he paused for long periods of time to listen to my words and reflect on what I had said. By the time I left the room, which was furnished with a comfortable couch and accented with décor reflective of his personal style, more than an hour had passed. If I were to add up the time that I had seen all three of my previous doctors together, that summation would not have been close to an hour. A sense of relief calmed my nervous stomach; I had been listened to and I had been heard.

Along with a homeopathic remedy for the anxiety I felt surrounding my symptoms, Doctor G prescribed to me a potassium supplement, as well as a few other holistic remedies. More importantly, he gave me a sense of hope.

"The body wants to heal itself, Kimberly. If you establish behaviors and habits that support your body's efforts to heal, you will see how powerful you truly are," his words lingered with me as I walked out the door.

I spent months searching for something, some doctor or some pill or some treatment, to fix me—to heal me. Out of all the commercials and advertisements that flooded my television and computer screen, I did not believe that there was not a convenient solution for my symptoms. After all, I lived in a society that made profits from quick fixes and thrived on the back of a gluttonous and bloated pharmaceutical industry. In college, a large portion of my peers were prescribed some sort of drug that allowed them to function on a day to day basis without having to really fix what was wrong. If I had followed my physician's recommendation to go see a psychiatrist, I too could have found a solution that I could swallow.

Had I known all along that there was not a quick fix to my problems? Had I ever been told that my body is a miraculous machine composed of intelligent cells that have a propensity for healing and renewal? Some say that we are born *tabula rasa* or as a "blank slate" and that all knowledge must come from perception and experience. In contrast, others believe Carl Jung's theory of the collective unconscious, which can be defined as a database of unconscious experiences, such as impulses and innate archetypes,

14

which are shared among beings of the same species. Was the real solution to my health crisis inside of my unconscious mind all along?

Within a week of visiting Doctor G, I began to feel relief. I woke up feeling better rested and felt less light-headed as the day progressed. My arms and legs tingled less and the immense weight that had been constantly crushing down on my chest began to lift. I slowly implemented some of the lifestyle changes that Doctor G had recommended. Hydrate more and drink less alcohol. Become more active and rest without distraction. Eliminate inflammatory agents from my diet, specifically gluten products and dairy products (essentially any type of food that could be referred to as a "product") and cook more wholesome meals.

Another week passed and I felt comfortable leaving my house to run simple errands as I began to find a sense of routine. Having more energy, I researched ways to further my knowledge on how to take back my health. I only just began to feel well again so I was terrified of allowing myself to slip back into sickness. Researching nutrition, I stumbled across the Institute for Integrative Nutrition™. I never imagined that I would begin a career as a Health Coach because the job seemed intimidating, but the idea of learning how to feed my body to nourish my own health seemed non-negotiable. The next day, I enrolled.

Attending the Institute for Integrative Nutrition opened my eyes and awakened my innate desire to thrive, to feel healthy and to be full of life. The concept of living authentically in alignment with my long-term goals and daily intentions consumed me. Over the course of the year, I began to implement all of the valuable knowledge that I was learning into my daily life and I started to heal. After graduating, I went on to become a board certified Holistic Health Practitioner with the American Association of Drugless Practitioners. I began to develop a personal yoga practice and study meditation as I worked to become a certified Hatha Yoga Teacher. Each day my passion for wellness grew. Each day I woke up and made the choice to live in wellness and abundance.

I discovered the value of living in the moment and facing my days with awareness. Living mindfully became more to me than something that I could read about.

It became my way of life.

Progress is The Process

You wake up and brush your teeth. Why? You have been brushing your teeth every morning since your mouth had teeth to be brushed. It's an important habit to form in order to maintain good oral hygiene. You don't debate whether or not to brush your teeth every morning. It has become a foundational part of your daily routine and is done without much thought. Like brushing your teeth, all habits are formed as a response to a particular need or situation and have a tendency of becoming involuntary.

Habits are formed through reinforcement—positive or negative—of a specific behavior on a consistent basis across a span of time. A lot of our fundamental habits are formed during the developmental stage of our lives when we are young.

Monkey, see. Monkey, do.

Some things in life must be involuntary for survival. Breathing is an involuntary action that is critical to sustaining life. The release of adrenaline when faced with a life threatening situation is involuntary and essential to avoid the threat of death. It is critical to look at your habits and evaluate how they impact your life and whether or not you are allowing these habitual automatic responses to take precedent over your conscious decision-making capacities. The only way to rewire your life and rework your patterns of behavior, negating the self-destructive habits that have become second nature, is to live in your body with awareness by occupying the present moment to make conscious choices.

In addition to studying creative writing and psychology in college, I studied philosophy. While all of my philosophy courses resonated with me, one course entitled "The Philosophy of the

Mind", helped changed the way I viewed human behavior. The curriculum reviewed the unresolved philosophical debate on whether animals are conscious beings and to what extent they possess thoughts, reason, and awareness. One of the philosophies studied throughout the curriculum was from Rene Descartes', a 17th century French philosopher; he maintained that animals lack both occurrent thought and reason. Animals, to philosophers like Descartes, were viewed as creatures that do not operate with awareness. Instead, they function robotically through reactionary patterns of behavior that are prompted by stimuli in their environment.

Whenever I left this philosophy class and began to go through my daily routine, I could not help but look around and feel as if my peers, and myself included, were becoming more robotic and less conscious of our choices; forgoing our ability to use thought and reason. We were sacrificing a life of awareness for the convenience of living through a series of cause and effect reactions. Rather than using thought and reason to overcome adversity or deal with daily situations, it seemed that this reactionary type of behavior had become a knee-jerk response. Like a doctor testing reflexes, an event hit one's life like a mallet to the knee and the person swung forward without hesitation into a reactionary response. Animals were more aligned with their relationship to their surroundings than human beings, who were stuck in the motions of a cause and effect cycle.

According to a study recorded by the Center for Disease Control in recent years, more than half of American adults have one or more health disorders directly related to lifestyle habits, meaning they fall under the categorization of having Multiple Chronic Conditions. More than half of the adults living in the United States allowed their habitual responses to hijack their health and negatively impact their lives. If you were to ask someone with diabetes if they like being diabetic, they would say do not like being diabetic. If you were to inform that same person of some simple lifestyle changes to manage or even reverse the symptoms associated with being a diabetic, it would be natural to assume that this person would desire the ability to help heal their bodies and be free of the associated limitations.

> "It seems, in fact, as though the second half of a man's life is made up of nothing, but the habits he has accumulated during the first half."
> –Fyodor Dostoyevsky

With the mounting pressures of our technologically advanced society, it is increasingly easy for one to resign themselves to living through a string of involuntary habits. There is work to be done and eating is viewed through terms of convenience rather than nutrition. Bills need to be paid and sleeping will not keep debt collectors at bay. Allowing one's self to become caught up in "the grind" and the stressors of the "real world" will result in one's living outside of the present moment, forcing one to revert to living through habitual behavioral responses. This pattern of behavior starts off as a coping mechanism and develops beyond our scope of introspective evaluation. When one feels overwhelmed by stressors, self-neglect, physical sickness, stress, depression, and apathy become prevalent. While it is encoded in our very DNA to strive for optimal health and wellness, we have somehow tricked ourselves into believing that there are "more important things" in life and that feeling less than our best is "normal".

Through the experiences I had with my own struggle for wellness, I realized that the only way to eliminate my destructive habits and eradicate my being from illness was to replace the old habits with new self-serving behaviors that were in alignment with the goals I had for my health and happiness. I chose to stop outsourcing my health; to stop waiting for a doctor to cure my body and start working to help my body heal itself. The key for establishing new habits that will support wellness and happiness is to live mindfully in the moment. Mindful living requires being present in whatever situation you are facing and making a conscious decision to handle the situation to best serve your health. It is critical, when taking back control of your health to be awake within your body, to occupy your being, and actively engage with all that is occurring inside of yourself and in your environment.

Mindful living cannot be surmised through one idea or achieved by doing one specific action. It is a machine composed of many moving parts, and each part of this machine must be optimally functioning both independently and harmoniously within the system. One cannot simply meditate and truly live mindfully. One cannot simply eat with intention and be in optimal physical shape. Like any machine, one part cannot work without the efficiency of the other. Your body cannot function without your mind, your mind cannot live without your body, and you cannot be a conscious being without having both a mind and body to occupy.

The intention of sharing my personal story and all that is to follow over the course of this book is to gift you with the tools that I have acquired to live a truly mindful life. Maybe you struggle with student loans. Maybe you have lived with the pain of a physical disease. Maybe you battle with depression. Whatever your struggle, whatever your pain, you have such an immense capacity to free yourself. You have the chance to awaken your life and you have the choice—each moment in every day—to choose health and happiness.

"If every day is an awakening, you will never grow old.
You will just keep growing."
-Gail Sheehy

You Can't Spell Revolution without **Evolution**

"Personal transformation can and does
have global effects. As we go,
so goes the world, for the world
is us. The revolution that will save the world
is ultimately a personal one."
-Marianne Williamson

Revolt, Recycle, Restart

For every point in history, there are moments that define culture and shape the future of the world. These moments are commonly defined as revolutions. If you search for the definition of the word *revolution*, you will find two different definitions. Merriam-Webster simply defines revolution as the following:

- **A sudden, extreme, or complete change in the way people live, work, etc.**

- **The action of moving around something in a path that is similar to a circle**

Under the more detailed version of the descriptions, you will read about the sudden and extreme changes that are classified under a social or cultural revolution. A revolution involves a shift in paradigms and a change in the fundamental views of a people. Pick any time period in human history and there will be discussion of one or many revolutions bridging gaps between generations.

When looking at a more detailed description of the second definition you will read about bodies, celestial or otherwise, moving on an axis around a fixed point and ending this cycle of momentum in the initial start place. Think of the planets revolving around the sun on their elliptical axis, staying true to their course and always winding up back where they started.

Although these two definitions of this one momentous word are rather different, viewed through comparison, they actually appear to be invariably linked. In the way that the Earth revolves around the Sun, the revolutions of humanity rotate around many of the same issues through time and across the globe. To shape the future, we must stop circling around in the patterns of the past and look inward to break the cycle. Unlike the planets that are fixed in their orbit, we can choose to end up in a place other than where we first began.

Imagine if you could impact the world just by becoming a healthier and happier version of your already remarkable self.

We have perfected the art of protesting against things, of reacting to the situations at hand. What we need to do instead is advocate for what we want and take preventative and proactive measures to achieve these goals. We become overwhelmed by the hefty list of all that needs to be changed in our lives so we tend to surrender to the idea that we cannot make any real change. Standing in the shadow of a massive tower of problems, we forget that there cannot be a shadow without the existence of a source of light—that we have the foresight to create our vision for a thriving world.

"Changing is not just changing the things outside of us. First of all we need the right view that transcends all notions including of being and non-being, creator and creature, mind and spirit. That kind of insight is crucial for transformation and healing."
-Thich Nhat Hanh

Think Outside the Box, Live Outside the Circle

A popular fable in Greek Mythology tells of Sisyphus, the cunning king of Corinth who cheated death. As punishment, the trickster king was sentenced to roll a boulder up a hill for the rest of eternity. Each time he reached the top, the boulder would roll back down to the bottom. Although the reason for this particular sentence remains a debate, the theme of fruitless labor as punishment is repetitive throughout mythology.

The pages of literature and of our history books alike exemplify this Sisyphus cycle on a loop. Empires were built and then collapsed. Civilizations rose to the top of the proverbial hill and inevitably rolled back down to the bottom. We can continue to push our hopes for a better world up this steep hill, over all of the obstacles we have established through the use of a redundant societal map, but we will continue to wind up in the valley of our past: staring up at the same hill that has always been blocking our capacity for growth.

The size of the boulder is set and the slope of the hill is fixed but our strategy for success is flexible; as human beings we have the neurological capacity to use reason and the aptitude to adjust to static circumstances. Unlike Sisyphus who was tragically stuck in a perceptive reality where time was "eternity", we live in a reality where, in relation to the progression of time, we evolve and overcome environmental conditions. Survival of a species requires adaptability but for our species to thrive *intentional* adaptations must be made consciously. We may not be able to immediately change our genetic makeup but we can create sustainable change for the future, one conscious decision at a time. We have come to the point in history where we can consciously impact the path of our own evolution.

In order to live outside of the circle, we must choose to think outside of the box—to revolutionize the societal landscape of the world through the effects of personal evolution. It is our duty as conscious beings to live in the light of awareness and to utilize all the tools at our disposal, therefore forcing sustainable change for the future. It is our duty as citizens of this shared planet to take responsibility for the impact that we have on our environment, on our global culture, and on our own bodies. We must stop outsourcing our health. We must stop expecting the next generation to work for change. We must stop blaming the institutions we continue to maintain through our apathetic participation; we must start enacting the change we wish to see.

We cannot build a road to a thriving collective future by navigating the old and outdated maps of our past. To establish optimal personal and global wellbeing, we must take responsibility as captains of our individual lives and as co-captains of the collective future.

How we interact with our immediate surroundings on a daily basis impacts the ever-evolving landscape of our home on Earth. The choices you make—from the food or food-like-products you chose to consume to the possessions you chose to surround yourself with to the career path you decide to embark upon—directly impacts your health and the health of our world at large. Through the practice of living with awareness and actively engaging with our daily routines, we can build stronger and more healthful patterns of behavior that will create an improved and sustainable overall personal and cultural wellbeing.

The development of eating a variety of locally sourced organic foods, the establishment of a morning routine that boosts energy and encourages mental clarity, and the cleansing and meditative practice of engaging in physical activity are a few of many ideas that will be explored in the upcoming pages. Borrowing from a variety of schools of thought it is the intention of this book to shed light on how you have the individual power, and responsibility, to wake up each day to make choices that will evolve your personal health and impact your immediate community as well as the global human body. Through the active and mindful occupation of our individual bodies, we will discover a deeper collective cognitive clarity.

Whether you have a desire to heal yourself of one or more chronic health conditions, to wake up with an abundance of energy and mental clarity, to overcome your struggle with managing your weight, or to liberate your life from the monotony of a shallow and repetitive daily routine—you have the capacity to find and establish permanent change. Our bodies are miraculous and complex mechanisms that continually work to maintain optimal health; we can consciously help our bodies heal by providing proper nourishment through physical nutrition and principal lifestyle practices.

I invite you to take this as a call to action, not to arm yourselves with weapons in the streets or to *protest* with signs and pickets but to arm yourself with conscious living in the environment of your daily lives and to *advocate for* personal growth and transformation.

> "I learned a long time ago the wisest
> thing I can do is be on my own side,
> be an advocate for myself
> and others like me."
> -Maya Angelou

Occupy Your Body

"Health is a state of complete harmony
of the body, mind and spirit.
When one is free from physical disabilities
and mental distractions,
the gates of the soul open."
-B.K.S. Iyengar

At the Corner of Cosmic and Corporeal

There was a time when the educated and literate people of the world held onto the belief that the sun revolved around the earth. Our planet, as well as our existence was at the center of the universe. This belief, like all beliefs, largely shaped human behavior. Through advancements of science, it came to be discovered that the sun was at the center of our solar system and we existed in only one of uncountable galaxies in the universe. Each galaxy contains billions, possibly hundreds of billions of stars. The number of stars in the expanse of the universe exceeds the scope of current human technology and is larger than any numerical value the human brain can conceptualize. Scientists estimated that there are around 100 octillian stars in the universe: to simplify, that number contains 29 zeros.

Stars are big burning balls of gas mostly composed of hydrogen and helium but also contain smaller amounts of heavier elements such as carbon, iron, nitrogen and oxygen. When the star expires, essentially running out of fuel, the elements that gave life to the star are released back into space and are recycled, creating the new life of another star. Similarly, the human body is composed of cells, and like the gaseous bodies of stars, the seemingly solid bodies of human beings are made of elements. The four major elements that compose the human body are hydrogen, oxygen, carbon, and nitrogen. The same elements that compose stars are the composition of the organic matter that occupies our

25

planet, and create the very body in which you are occupying this very moment. Our existence on this planet was birthed from the violent and magnificent death of stars.

We are made from star dust and have a fundamental connection to the vast universe that houses us. We live at the corner of cosmic and corporeal; occupying the space between the mineral sediments below our feet and the endless ether above our heads.

Without being an astronomer, biologist, or mathematician, the importance of this cosmic connection can be appreciated. This comparison of stars to cells—the cosmic to the corporeal—brings to light the ability to think critically and, to view what we see with our eyes through a scope of deeper understanding. Stars are gasses and elements, fusion and gravity, pressure and energy. Human beings are tissues and elements, fluids and organs, mind and emotion, energy and matter. When thinking about our own bodies, the path to physical wellness starts with our willingness to look deeper into understanding than what can be seen through the limited lens of the human eye.

Whether it is among the stars or on the landscapes of our planet, life is created from the magic of chemical reactions. A star is fueled by the fusion that occurs at its core; the energy produced from the chemical changes that occur when the element hydrogen is transformed to the element helium. Inside the human body, many chemical processes are needed to produce the energy that fuels our lives.

The moment that we place food into our mouths, the digestion process begins, turning food into fuel. The salivary enzymes in our mouths, helped out by the physical action of chewing, kick off the chemical process. Our stomachs host enzymes and acids that further break down what we have eaten. From there, the pancreatic enzymes and bacteria in the intestines take over. The output of energy is dependent of the efficiency of these chemical responses and therefore, the food we choose to ingest will either aid or exhaust our digestive system. Whereas stars, plants, and bacteria do not have free will to influence the process of creating life-sustaining energy, humans do.

By having a choice in what we eat, we have the ability to directly impact the life sustaining systems that provide our bodies with energy. If you have ever heard the sayings, "trust your gut" or "follow your gut," there is a more literal meaning behind these words than one might initially infer. Our gut, also known as the enteric nervous system, or what scientists have named "the second brain," is a nine meter long tube containing sheaths of neurons within the walls of its lining. The author of *The Second Brain,* an expert in the field of neurogastronenterology, Michael Gershon, estimates that the number of neurons within the gut is around 100 million.

With growing exploration on the role played by the second brain, more urgent information is being discovered on how our gut has the capacity to send messages to our brain in addition to facilitating our immune system. The gut's purpose extends far beyond acting as a center where chemical reactions and digestion occurs; it reaches into the very fiber of our emotions and wellbeing. What we eat does not only build our bodies on a physical level—creating our cells, blood, and tissues—but what we eat has a direct impact on who we are and how we feel on a day to day basis.

"The body is your temple. Keep it pure
and clean for the soul to reside in."
-B.K.S. Iyengar

The Neural Pathway Highway

Water has the capacity to shape landscapes by carving paths through bodies of land, many that we have established our homes on. The water erodes the land, wearing away at the surface to form lasting impressions upon the landscape, creating rivers and streams. Our thoughts behave like water: freely flowing out from our brain and eroding away at our biology to build specific paths of behavior. If we are not mindful of what direction we allow our thoughts to flow, the landscape of our lives can dramatically change.

Our perceptions, beliefs, and thoughts are powerful tools that either enhance or inhibit our lives. If you view yourself as a capable and empowered individual, chances are that you will be willing to work hard to achieve your life's goals. If you believe that you are undeserving and inferior to others, there is a strong chance that you will live in the shadow of your insecurities. What we think directly impacts the choices we make on a fundamental level in our daily lives.

Every choice that we make is based on our pervious experiences, projected anxieties, and belief patterns which we desperately hold onto. We have narrowed our scope of perception to see only the path we have been on, preventing us from a new path; one where our life begins to flow toward realization of total wellness and lasting contentment.

Have you ever found meaning in a situation that occurred by coincidence, that you had previously foreseen, as if your thoughts somehow manifested a certain life experience or event? The term for this type of phenomena was coined by Carl Jung, a psychologist who began his exploration of the human psyche under the guidance of Sigmund Freud. Synchronicity shows how powerful our thoughts, conscious or unconscious, can be in relation to our perceptive realities. From wherever our thoughts flow, they wind up engraining a path to a certain event in our life that is meaningful.

New Age philosophies have adopted this concept and formulated a belief where one has the capacity to manifest a specific perceptive reality. Through your thoughts you attract certain events, people, and circumstances into your life, like a magnet to metal. Where your thoughts flow, your life will go. Interestingly, neuroscientists have been studying the power behind the energetic waves produced by our thoughts and how these waves interact with our perceptive realities. Similar to a sound wave physically interacting with the atmosphere, thought waves interact with the space in which we occupy.

Our thoughts have the capacity to bridge the separation between our self and our environment, acting as a mirror to reflect our inner world onto our outer world. Over recent years, many biologists and doctors have taken an interest in the power of thought waves and have begun researching how our thoughts impact our own internal environment in addition to our external.

When we have an emotional response to stimuli, or have trained our bodies to live in the cause and effect mode cited earlier in the book, the brain uses neural pathways to release certain hormones that cause certain reactions. Whether adrenaline or dopamine is released depends on the emotional response that follows the reaction to an event. The different hormones released in the body will cause different chemical reactions that then establish different biological conditions in the body's environment.

Researchers are studying how the biological environment we create through our thoughts and emotional responses affects our genetic composition, and our health. This field of genetic study, known as Epigenetics, is causing researchers to believe that we can control which genes are expressed inside of our bodies—just like turning a light switch on and off in a room.

The idea that our thoughts can either make us sick or help us heal is being proven through scientific research. This research is disproving the belief that our health is at the mercy of our DNA; we have the power to help heal our bodies and prevent diseases by establishing a healthy environment for our bodies to thrive in. We are in the position to train our brains to build healthy emotional responses to the circumstances of our outer world in order to build a thriving environment for our inner world.

"The moment you change your perception,
is the moment you rewrite the chemistry of your body."
-Dr. Bruce Lipton

The same way that we say **you are what you eat**, we should also say **you are what you think**. What we eat builds our cells and tissues while what we think builds the environment that will either support healthy or unhealthy traits to be expressed from those cells. We have the power to directly impact our chemical biology, our health, and our wellbeing.

Fuel for the Journey

A popular analogy made between the human body and cars asks whether or not a person would want to put the most efficient fuel in their vehicle. Of course, the owner of a car does not want to ruin their investment and wants to place the best fuel inside of their car. The person is then forced to consider whether or not they want to place the best fuel inside their body. While this analogy forces people to understand that food is fuel, an even deeper comparison can be made.

Take into consideration that the car does not only have an engine that requires fuel but also a computer system that operates the car's engine. Your body is much like the car in the sense that your body is both an engine that requires fuel and a computer-like mind that operates the engine of your body. Your body and a car's computer are both highly efficient machines that require data to be entered in order to produce output. If the data that you put into your computer is corrupt, for example with a virus, the computer will become infected and your vehicle will not operate. If the data being placed into your body—the DNA of the food you allow into your digestive tract and the ideas and thoughts you allow into your mind—is corrupt, the body will be unable to properly process the data and your body will not operate. Both the hardware and the software must be properly handled in order for the vehicle to run, the computer to operate, and your body and mind to thrive.

When considering the food you eat, or the fuel for your journey, you must consider how it will interact with your body on a cellular level. When you look at an apple, consider that you are not eating the redness of the apple or the sweetness of the apple but you are ingesting the genetic data of the apple; you are enjoying what looks like an apple to your eyes and tastes like an apple to your mouth, but you are digesting the minerals and nutrients that compose the apple. When you strip away the

30

sensory experiences of an apple, you are left with the raw data that makes the apple an apple and that will transform, through the chemical processes of your body, into your cells, fluids, tissues, and organs.

When you look at food-like products with this critical lens, the ingredients that make the product become questionable. When looking at a picture of a food-like product on a box, you are ingesting the data through your sensory perceptions and the data becomes fragmented into aesthetics, texture, taste, and smells. The image on the box may look like food, represent the idea of food, and maybe it tastes like food, but once you begin to read the "nutrition facts" and ingredients, you realize that the contents within the packaging are not actually food.

The ingredients, or chemical data, of the food-like products are not the natural data (meaning whole and complete nutritious food DNA) that your body requires to efficiently build your cells, fluids, tissues, and organs. Eating processed food-like products is like trying to place a square block in a round hole; the idea of a shape is present but the structure of the shape is incorrect. If you try to input incomplete and fragmented data into your computer, the operating system will not be able to properly function and process the data in a way that is efficient and complete.

By randomly ingesting fragmented pieces of DNA from our food sources that have been extracted or replicated to make a new type of food-product, our bodies are not capable of properly processing this DNA data in a way that efficiently builds a complete body operating system.

In a similar manner, the computer like mind that controls the physical structure of one's body must receive nourishing data that promotes functionality and optimization. If one is host to corrupted streams of information, the operating system of the body cannot function efficiently. When a new update is available for the operating system on your phone, you must clear old data in order to make room for the new and improved data. It is important to review what thoughts and beliefs no longer serve our body's system in order to let go of these outdated beliefs and make

31

room for continual growth.

Because we have a tendency to hold onto old beliefs and behavioral patterns as a means of familiarity and comfort in an ever-evolving world, we limit our growth and negatively impact the efficiency of our body's capacity to promote self-healing and authentic wellness. Your thoughts are a critical part of your body's processing center and you have control over what information flows throughout the system and what information gets deleted.

In the same manner that it is essential to fuel your body with whole, natural and nourishing food that contains the essential minerals and vitamins to build healthy cells in your body, it is critical to fuel your mind with the wholesome, natural and nourishing thoughts that build a healthy environment, so that your body's cells grow in a way that promotes health and well-being.

If you are holding onto incomplete thoughts such as, "I am not good enough" or "I do not deserve to invest in my health," thoughts that fragment how you are a perfect (meaning complete) being of body, mind and spirit, you will be held back from growing inward and expressing a more complete version of your being. Deciding to literally digest thoughts that remind us of the totality of our beings, such as, "My body creates a healthy environment that promotes growth for my mind and spirit," will support the simultaneous evolution of our bodies with our minds and in alignment with our spirits.

Once one's body is operating in the most efficient way possible, one has the capacity to exceed physical and emotional limitations in order to flourish in the more profound ways of life, such as the expansion of individual consciousness and the growth of a strong interconnectedness between all sentient beings.

The bottom line is that your body wants to maintain a balanced and healthful physical, emotional, and spiritual environment. You have the ability to bring awareness into your life by making the choices to eat whole foods and to think health-promoting thoughts. Eating mindfully and being conscious of your beliefs and behavior patterns can be achieved through manageable daily steps. The key to finding balance is to be mindful of all the elements necessary for nourishment by taking them in smaller more digestible steps. The next part of this section gives practical tips on how to begin the process of mindfully living in your body to promote health and wellness.

Fuel Economy for Your Body
How to Eat Mindfully and Occupy Your Body

Designer vs. Discount:
Within the world of fashion, the more expensive an item, the more desirable that item becomes. Inversely, within the world of food, the cheaper the products the more desirable the product becomes. We have confused our priorities when it comes to our physical appearance and our internal needs. We cannot have a designer appearance on a discounted diet. Eating to support a healthy body does not require draining your 401k but it does require an awareness and a desire to invest more into how you feel than how you are perceived. When it comes to your food, buying and eating habits, ask yourself the following questions:

1. <u>Does the majority of what I eat come pre-packaged in colorful plastic or cardboard?</u>
    - If it doesn't come wrapped in colorful package, it is probably produce and you should consider purchasing it. While local organic produce is generally better for a variety of reasons than non-organic grocery store produce, purchasing produce over packaged goods is desirable. Many pre-packaged foods are more product than food. A healthy body requires proper fuel and we are designed to digest real whole foods and not chemically engineered food-like products.

2. <u>Does the food that I eat and do the restaurants where I dine have commercials advertising a low price as a desirable feature?</u>
    - If your food has its own commercial, it is probably a food-like product and should be avoided. When it comes to what we eat, the concepts of cheap and convenient are not ideal. If you are what you eat, do you want to be cheap or do you want to be priceless?

3. Do you recognize all the ingredients listed on the nutrition label? How long is the list of ingredients?
   - Read the labels on the food products you do purchase. When it comes to purchasing premade foods, the shorter the label the better. Avoid foods with labels that have a long list of ingredients. If you do not recognize the listed ingredients, look them up on the internet (you are more than likely to have a phone with internet, where there are a ton of downloadable applications that will clarify the ingredient for you), you may be very surprised to learn what the ingredient is, where it is derived, and how it has been shown to interact with the human body.

Eat With Intention

There is a reason why grandma's chicken soup was the go-to fix when you were sick as a kid. Grandma prepared that soup with love and intention, she was mindful of which ingredients were used to make this magical healing remedy. It is important that as individuals, responsible for our own health, we prepare our meals with the intention of nourishing our bodies.

Try This Exercise, on a separate sheet of paper. Make a list of what your diet looks like on an average day:

- ➤ Breakfast:_____
- ➤ Lunch:_____
- ➤ Dinner:_____
- ➤ Snacks:_____
- ➤ Water Intake (in ounces): _____

Now take a moment and right below this current Daily Diet example, write what you think an ideal diet would look like for your body and lifestyle:

- ➤ Breakfast:_____
- ➤ Lunch:_____
- ➤ Dinner:_____
- ➤ Snacks:_____
- ➤ Water Intake (in ounces): _____

Below this Ideal Diet, take a moment and write what your intentions are when you choose what to eat.

Is it your intention to get something, anything, in your stomach before you fly out the door in a rush for work?

Is it your intention to lose weight in a quick and convenient way?

OR, is it your intention to eat the foods that will properly provide your body with fuel and nourish your body throughout the day, giving you ample energy and allowing you to feel well?

Reflecting on the intentions you set brings awareness to your focus, or lack of, on what impact the food will have on your body and on your day.

Now, take a moment to blend your current Daily Diet with your intentions from your Ideal Diet. This way of eating should be something you feel is realistic and comfortable for your body. Every individual has different nutritional needs. Listen to your body's needs and set the intention to fulfill these needs in an accessible way.

> Breakfast:_____
> Lunch:_____
> Dinner:_____
> Snacks:_____
> Water Intake (in ounces):_____

Enjoy the process of cooking. Remember the intention to nourish your body with the essentials that it needs in order to thrive. Cooking meals does not need to be time consuming and intimidating. Start with basic things that you enjoy and look up ways to incorporate dishes and ingredients you may never have tried. It is a fun process of self-discovery that will enable you to experience the benefits of having a diverse diet. This will also help you eliminate the old habit of depending on others to provide your meals for you.

Cook once and eat multiple times. Begin to develop a system of meal preparation that is time savvy and allows you to enjoy convenience and quality. This practice saves money as well as time. Preparing simple side dishes or lunches ahead of time to be enjoyed throughout the week will prevent you from scrambling last minute to figure out a meal on the fly.

For more on developing a personal strategy to better fuel your body and for fun recipe ideas, feel free to visit my website at www.unearthyourwarrior.com.

Eat Without Distraction

- Taste is amplified by sight and smell, so pausing to appreciate your food using all the senses will develop mindfulness and help you savor the meal.
- DO NOT watch television or participate in other mindless distractions while eating. By not allowing yourself the time to focus on enjoying your meal, you increase the chances of overeating and this can limit your gut's ability to signal when to stop.
- Make sure to chew your food. Taking the time to chew your food thoroughly will aid the digestive process and create an awareness of how much you are consuming.

Outside of the Kitchen

- Set aside blocks of time in your week to perform physical activity:
  If you do not like the gym, functional exercise can be just as beneficial. Go on a walk. Begin a yoga practice. Start a garden. Walk your dog.
- Stretch throughout the day: If you have a job that requires sitting for extended periods of time, take a short break every 60 to 90 minutes to stand up and stretch. Our lymphatic system, the system that helps to rid our body of

toxins, does not have a self-circulating mechanism. For example, our circulatory system has the heart to pump blood, but the lymphatic system requires physical activity to move lymph throughout the body and eliminate the wastes that keep us feeling lethargic and lackluster. Taking breaks to tend to your body will increase productivity rather than taking up precious work time. When you feel good, you will work with more clarity and tenacity.

Simple Stretches:

Sit upright in your chair and evenly distribute your weight on both sit bones. Engage your core by drawing the navel back and up toward the spine. Allow your shoulder blades to drop down and back, engaging them as a part of your back body. Keep your arms at your sides. As you take a deep inhale through your nose, sweep your arms up and around so your palms touch above your head. Gaze up at your hands. Exhale out through the nose and lower your arms back down towards your sides. Repeat this process a few times. Add in stretching the side of your body by interlocking your fingers once your palms touch above the head and stretch to the right, to the left and to the back.

Staying in the same upright position, take a big inhale through the nose and on the exhale, drop your right ear toward your right shoulder. Inhale your head back to center. Exhale and drop your chin down toward your chest, interlock your fingers and place your palms on the back of your neck at the base of your head, gently pressing with some resistance. Release your hands. Inhale and lift the chin back to center. On the next exhale, drop your left ear towards your left shoulder. Inhale and lift your chin back to center. Repeat this simple neck stretch a few times.

The stretches that you engage in for brief periods of time throughout the day do not need to be complicated or intensive. The purpose is to get the blood flowing, the lymph moving, and to prevent lactic acid build up in the muscles.

- Drink plenty of water:

    More than half of the human body is water. In a world where some people have access to unlimited water, chronic dehydration is a huge problem that is affiliated with many chronic health conditions. The more water you drink the less sugary beverages you will consume. A good rule of thumb, endorsed by many doctors and health experts alike, is to take your body weight, cut it in half, and consume that number in ounces of water daily.

    For example: 130lbs/2 = 65ounces of water. It is good to have a water goal in order to make an effort to drink water.

Water Bottle Trick:

    Purchase a reusable BPA free water bottle of your choosing. Know how many ounces the water bottle contains and how many ounces you are trying to consume a day. Get colorful rubber bands. Apply one rubber band to the water bottle in the beginning of the day for how many refills are needed in order to reach your water consumption goal. Every time you finish the bottle, remove one of the rubber bands so you know how many refills are left.

    For example: 130lbs/2 = 65 ounces of water. One 16oz water bottle would need to be filled 4 times in order to reach the goal of 65 ounces. Place 4 different rubber bands on the bottle and remove one after each refill. This is a very simple way to build mindfulness and keep an awareness of how much water you are consuming daily.

    If you feel that water is boring and tasteless, there are awesome ways to flavor your water naturally without adding sugars. Get a reusable water bottle or even a larger jug, cut up some of your favorite fruits and herbs, place them in the bottle with purified water and allow them to sit overnight in the fridge. The next day, your water will be packed with flavor and packed with the nutrients from the fruits and herbs!

* If you have been diagnosed with a health condition or are currently taking any medication, it is important to consult with your doctor on how much water is right for you.

Meditation in Motion

In March of 2014, the results of a study done by clinicians at Johns Hopkins University, was published in *JAMA Internal Medicine*. The study was on the impact of meditation and mindfulness on psychological stressors. The results suggested that mindfulness and meditation can help to manage and ease psychological stressors such as depression, anxiety, and even pain. Various studies across the broad spectrum of health and science research are showing that meditation is a useful tool to improve overall wellbeing and life quality.

Developing a meditation practice is a critical way to bring awareness to your body and how you feel living inside of your body. Yoga, even though it is a physical practice involving movement, is a meditative practice. Through yoga, the practitioner learns how to observe their bodies with awareness and without judgment. The Yogi or Yogini learns how to position their body into proper alignment for each posture as they mindfully flow from one pose into the next.

Yoga also involves an acute focus on breath awareness. Deep and mindful breathing allows the mind to quiet, increases the flow of oxygen, and activates rest-and-digest mode through the parasympathetic nervous system. As a yoga teacher and practitioner, I highly recommend developing a morning or nighttime yoga practice to bring your body in closer alignment with your health goals.

For those who may not be ready to begin a yoga practice or have limited mobility, engaging in simple meditations are a great way to get acquainted with these concepts. A meditation to build mindfulness within your body could be something as simple as the following. Read this meditation and then allow yourself some time to experience it before moving on in the book:

Find a quiet space in your environment where you feel comfortable and uncluttered. Sit up tall, and ground down into your sit bones while lifting upwards through the center of your head. Set the intention to create length within the spine.

Engage your pelvic floor by drawing your navel up and back; keep your abdominal muscles active. Allow the shoulders to drop down and back, away from the ears so you can elongate the neck. Close your eyes and begin to take deliberate and deep breathes in and out through the nose. Allow the silence to surround you as you drop your awareness deep down into your body. Whenever a thought arises, acknowledge this thought and then release it, as if it were a cloud floating by in the atmosphere of your mind. The more you try to fight off thoughts, the tougher it will be to detach from them.

Focusing on the breath, imagine a warm glowing white light begin to wash over your body with each inhale and exhale. Allow this light to start at the base of your feet and slowly flow up your legs, over your core, and up into your heart.

Imagine this white light is healing any pains or aches that may be stored in your muscles, tissues and bones. Physically feel the warmth of this light as it caresses and heals your body. Allow the light to swell and gather in your heart. Feel the light radiate out from your heart, sending immense and unconditional self-love to every cell in your body. Inhale. Exhale.

Allow the light to wash up past the throat and up into the forehead, where it rests right between the eyebrows in the third eye. Allow the light to warm your face and bring an illuminating clarity to your mind.

Finally allow this light to leave your body through the crown of your head; taking with it any and all discomfort or pain and leaving your body to feel open, calm and restored.

Take a moment before allowing your eyes to flutter open and returning to your surroundings.

At first, you may find meditation a difficult practice to begin. Every time you engage in meditation, you will find it less and less challenging. Beginning a yoga practice with a teacher to help guide you through meditations, or even listening to guided meditations found on the internet, will help you begin to develop a strong exploration of your own body and mind. If you are willing and dedicated, you will discover that all you need for an abundantly happy and healthy life is already within you.

"So what is a good meditator? The one who meditates."
– Allan Lokos

Affirmations for Your Body

Affirmations can be powerful tools when it comes to reminding ourselves of important truths that we often forget. When we allow ourselves to get caught up in the redundancy of daily activities, which may not make us feel our best, we tend to forget that we deserve to feel our best at each and every moment.

Taking the time to implement these affirmations into your daily life will help to keep you in touch with the intentions for your health and happiness. Yoga practitioners practice affirmations during meditation known as mantras.

Whether you desire to practice mantras in meditation or write affirmations to hang up in visible sight on your desk, here are a few affirmations about how you live in a powerful and miraculous body:

❖ I accept and love my body unconditionally.

❖ My body is a beautiful and powerful machine that works hard to bring balance and health into my life.

❖ I am capable of keeping my body healthy and happy. I am in control of how I care for my body.

❖ My body is a beautiful home in which my soul resides. I have love and respect for my body.

❖ I accept myself where I am and know that I have the power to grow.

❖ I choose to occupy my body with intention and awareness. I choose to live fully inside of my body with mindfulness.

Occupy Your Now

"Realize deeply that the present moment is all you have. Make the NOW the primary focus of your life."
-Eckhart Tolle, *The Power of Now: A Guide to Spiritual Enlightenment*

You Have A Past

Every day you wake up in the morning, you wake up as you; there is recognition of self and identity. You wake up in your bed, in your clothing, in your home, and you stand up to face a day that you have planned in your life. How do you know all of the information that makes you who you are? Your memories of the past are a trail of breadcrumbs that lead you to your future. You wake up and think to yourself, "I grew up in my home town with my parents and siblings; I had all of these experiences that have led me to be the person I am this morning. I have a name, an occupation and an identity."

If you woke up without any memories of whom you were the day before, of where you were the day before and where you were going the day after, it would be fair to assume that you would feel an abrupt and acute sense of panic and confusion. Without any attachment to the person you once were or the person you aspire to grow to become, you would be detached, disoriented, and directionless.

Our memories are crucial to building our identity. Our past experiences are the tracks to which we cling in order to propel ourselves forward. It is important to use these past memories and experiences to build a sense of self: to find a moral compass and discover unique skills, to acquire knowledge and grow from mistakes, and to take pride in one's successes.

However, there are times when we find ourselves trapped in the past—we get glued down to our prior experiences and are kept from moving forward. When we find ourselves caught in the past, bound to the emotions and beliefs of a certain event or experience, we cannot be open to the growth that comes from creating new experiences.

We have a tendency to feel comforted by the familiar, whether good or bad, because we have made a habit of resisting change. Living in the past does not serve your life in the present moment; instead, it prevents you from moving towards the future.

A balance can be found between the familiar story of our past, which we consistently tell ourselves, and the unknown plot development of the next page in our book. It is important to realize that you *have a past* but you are not defined by your past. When we choose to bring our past with us, it becomes impossible to live in the present moment because we are too focused on holding onto the person that we were in one precise instance surrounded by specifically set circumstances.

Although your mind has a very static sense of self which you have come to identify as your personality, in your three dimensional reality, you are susceptible to varying circumstances and surroundings. The only way to be truly content in the moment is to let go of any preconceived notions of self and to be open to growth and adaptations based on what events, circumstances and surroundings present themselves within each moment.

Think about your favorite story as a child, maybe it was the book that a parent read to you before bed or the first chapter book you read on your own. Reflect on why you loved that book.

Was it the beautiful illustrations?
Did you love the whimsical setting or the funny characters?
Did you admire the main character's bravery or charming talents?

If you were to purchase a copy of this favorite childhood book and reread it in the same manner as you once did, the story would be the same, but you would not. You have grown over a span of time. The person you are in the present moment is not the same as the child you were in the moments that have passed. Maybe you would find new reasons to love this childhood book or maybe you would be too disconnected to even see what in this story fascinated you in the first place.

As we grow and evolve, so does our taste in food, music and clothing. Our desire for certain pleasures and our aversions to certain pains become more refined and acute. So why is it that we are not capable of letting go of previous events that no longer connect with the person we are in this moment? You are not the character in your childhood story book.

You are capable of growing far beyond the limitations of the simpler language and ideas that once constructed your world. If you would not wear the clothes you once wore as a teenager, then why wear the identity of the person you were when you were hurt by a loved one or when you were presented with a certain obstacle.

"Experience is not what happens to you; it's what
you do with what happens to you."
-Aldous Huxley

In the same way that a snake sheds its skin or that a hermit crab outgrows its shell, the human body has cells that are constantly dying and regenerating. The human body's skin cells regenerate every 7 days, the cells of the human skeleton are replaced about every 7 years, and a cut will heal on average over the course of 2 weeks. Your body is constantly rebuilding, adapting, and renewing. You are capable of using this same concept in relation to your habits, belief systems, reactionary responses, and your sense of self. While there will always be certain characteristics that will remain unchanged about who you are—and for good reason—you have the choice of renewing your life on a daily basis.

Releasing the past does not involve forgetting where you came from, what experiences created your life, or who may have hindered or helped your development; it involves recognizing all of these things, but choosing to leave them behind you as you evolve and grow. Rather than waking up in your bed every morning attached to the emotions and challenges of yesterday, you can make the choice to face the opportunities of today with an open mind and a renewed sense of self.

In the way that we collect materialistic goods, we have become hoarders of experiences. We are attached to the ideas, feelings and emotions that were associated with a particular event or past experience. The only way to live in the moment and find freedom from the limitations of the past is to practice non-attachment.

The idea of living without attachment to the ideas and experiences that have identified and comforted us for so long is frightening. It was always scary as a child, letting go of the edge of the pool to swim out into the deep end or removing the training wheels from your bike, but the fear was only temporary and our growth was transcendent.

Living without attachment to our conditioned emotions, beliefs, and identity constructs is a skill that must be practiced. One must wake up every day and make the conscious decision to let go of what limits them as the person they used to be; instead, one must be open to embrace the unknown future, which will unleash the potential for who they can become.

There is A Future

Falling asleep at night can sometimes be a chore; in the space between processing our chores of the day and quieting our minds for sleep, our anxieties make themselves known. Suddenly, our mind becomes clogged with lists of tasks that need to be performed, of bills that need to be paid, and of obligations that must be fulfilled. The idea of *tomorrow* becomes the nightmare of today. Sometimes the notion of *tomorrow* isn't just about the upcoming 24 hours; our minds are worrying about events that may occur days, weeks or months from the current moment.

Eventually, thinking about the future becomes a burdened weight on our mind, rather than the uplifting idea that we are graced with the opportunity to experience more joy and happiness. Your stomach begins to churn thinking about the possible outcomes of a future event and your body begins to have an adverse reaction to the very thought of something that may or may not happen. Regardless of the fact that you are not currently experiencing a certain set of circumstances, your body feels sick with anxiety and your mind becomes overwhelmed.

Allowing the anxiety of your future to dictate your physical and emotional state in the present moment is like giving up your real life to live within a hologram or virtual reality. The events that are causing you distress are not immediate or real but instead they are projections of possibilities. Choosing to experience the world from this projected and imaginary mindset, takes you out of the present. Living in this future mindset causes stress and damage to your current physical and emotional wellbeing. Even if the stressors are not real, your mind processes the anxiety of these projected future possibilities as if they were in the here and now.

While it is essential for one's wellbeing to prepare to the best of one's ability for the future, such as having money saved for emergencies or planning ahead for one's retirement, it is detrimental to one's wellbeing to live each moment in anticipation of the next. You *have a future* but you are not defined by your future.

If you spend all of your time preparing for the endless amount of possibilities that may or may not arise in your life then you are missing out on the current experiences that you are supposed to be absorbing in order to grow and evolve. The best way to prepare for what is to come in your future is to live with awareness and authenticity in the moment that you currently occupy.

Although it may seem counterintuitive when viewed from a lens of logic, the only way to be prepared for the unknown future is to practice living with awareness in the present. The idea of practicing spontaneity may seem like an oxymoron, but it is critical to living a life full of joy and wellbeing. If you are living with expectations for the outcome of future events, you are limiting yourself only to those outcomes and you are closing yourself off the possibilities you did not predict.

You may also be setting yourself up to experience disappointment and frustration by allowing yourself to prematurely make an emotional attachment to a specific outcome you have not yet, and may never, experience. When you choose to live without expectation, you are opening yourself up to have an authentic and unbiased reaction to the endless possibilities of the future.

"A journey is a person in itself; no two are alike.
And all plans, safeguards, policing, and coercion are fruitless. We find
that after years
of struggle that we do not take a trip;
a trip takes us."
-John Steinbeck

Despite a future event being a fictitious scenario created in the mind, the damage to the physical body that comes from stress and anxiety is very real. Stressful situations place the body in fight-or-flight mode where the stress hormones norepinephrine (noradrenaline) and epinephrine (adrenaline) which increase ones heart rate and blood flow to the skeletal and muscular systems of the body.

When all of our energy is being poured into our fight-or-flight responses the rest of our body suffers from a lack of energy and our lifestyle begins to suffer from this disruptive physical imbalance. During this stress response, because so much of the body's energy is being used to react for survival, your brain's capacity to think critically becomes limited. You are literally limiting your ability to creatively solve a situation or overcome a specific circumstance by allowing your body to feel stressed.

Evolutionarily, the longest surviving species on this earth have adapted and evolved without making long "To Do" lists or staying awake at night anxiously anticipating the outcome of their business presentation the next day. They adapted by authentically reacting to unpredictable circumstances that occurred at random and without warning. They spontaneously evolved without thought or logic.

Being open to all future possibilities allows for a more proactive response and enables unanticipated growth, which may exceed beyond the preconditioned limitations imposed by trying to predict the future. Letting go of your future is the best way to find it.

Referring back to the analogy that you must let go of your past story to freely move forward in life, you must also let go of the expectations you have for your future story. When writing a novel, the writer may have a preset destiny in mind for a specific character. However, if the writer does their job in building this character a believable life and personality, the character begins to take on a life of their own; therefore, the character has authentic reactions to the story line that may have been unforeseen and unintended by the writer.

Imagine that your life is a novel and you are the writer. You may have one type of future in mind for yourself, but once you begin to act authentically in the moment, living free of attachment to expectations your future will take on a life of its own. By surrendering your expectations for the future you become more content with what is to come than you originally expected.

You Are the NOW

When it comes to your health, living in the present moment is non-negotiable. In order to live fully present in the *now*, you must challenge your current relationship with time. If you live your life as if time is fixed on a linear path—past, present, future—you are limiting yourself to exist only in that mindset. You will constantly be stuck inbetween your past and future; feeling squeezed by what has happened and pressured by what is to come.

When you challenge the idea that your life is like waiting in a very long line, you begin to realize that you are left with the spot in which you currently stand. There will be no rush to get to the front of the line and no constant looking over your shoulder to see how far you have come, you will feel contentment standing in the space that you currently occupy.

The phrase, "time flies when you're having fun" expresses how one's perception of time changes in relation to how one is living throughout the day. When we are enjoying an activity and are fully engaged in what we are doing, time seems to disappear. On the other hand, when we are sitting through an activity we find painstaking, time seems to drag on endlessly. Our mood and emotional state is generally dependent on how we are interacting with time and how we choose to perceive time throughout the day.

When we feel overwhelmed with tasks and live with stress, our day escapes us. We feel as if there is not enough time to get everything done, but we also feel as if our days are never-ending. Our bodies begin to feel the pressure of this stress and we become exhausted, drained of energy, fatigued, nauseous, and foggy-headed. Our immune system begins to wear down and our chances of becoming sick are increased.

Whether we feel as if our incomplete tasks of the past are on our heels or our future worries are closing in, we allow ourselves to live outside of the present moment leaving our body's physical and emotional wellbeing at the mercy of our own perceived stresses and pressures.

In stark contrast, when we are actively engaged in the present moment we allow our mind to process events and information as it is presented to us; this lets our body use the part of our brain that creatively solves problems and is capable of critical thinking. Not only does this stop the physical stress response from occurring, it also forces our mind to focus on what is happening presently.

When we live inside of the moment and keep our mind focused on what is coming to us as we receive it, we can literally digest the experience in a way that benefits our body—physically, mentally, and emotionally—and a sense of balance can be maintained.

When we live in the past or the future we are having a second hand experience; it is comparable to listening to a friend tell a story about a life experience they had. Living in this mindset, we prevent ourselves from authentically experiencing something real by only experiencing the ideas and thoughts of an event. Allowing our mind to process information in the present moment allows us to feel more vibrant with energy because we are having a direct life experience; we are having a genuine physical, emotional, and spiritual response in real time.

> "Write it on your heart that every day is the best
> day in the year."
> -Ralph Waldo Emerson

The autonomic nervous system, which is responsible, for our body's automatic operations, consists of two systems. One system is the sympathetic nervous system that is responsible for our Fight vs. Flight mode of survival. Stemming from our "reptilian brain," the oldest part of our brain, the sympathetic nervous system was essential for survival during the beginning stages of human evolution. When we live in the past or future we resign ourselves to react to situations from this part of our brain and we forfeit our ability to problem solve using reason, creativity and understanding.

When faced with a stressor, the sympathetic nervous system releases the stress hormones norepinephrine and epinephrine, also known as noradrenaline and adrenaline. When released into the blood stream, these hormones stimulate blood flow to the skeletal and muscular systems preparing the body for a physical response to the stressor. This chemical reaction made sense when our ancestors were faced with running from a predator or facing prey during a hunt. However, in our modern age the stressors we face do not tend to involve running from predators or fighting for our lives.

A constant release of stress hormones into our system inflicts serious damage onto our bodies and, ultimately, within our lives.

The autonomic nervous system is responsible for maintaining our body's homeostasis. Overworking this system makes it harder for our body to stay balanced. Health conditions related to stress range from heart conditions to gastrointestinal to psychological. The good news is that many of these conditions are preventable and some are reversible.

When we live mindfully in the moment we allow our bodies to activate the parasympathetic nervous system which allows our body to enter rest and digest mode. While in rest and digest mode our muscles relax, our heart rate drops, and our digestive enzymes are released.

The parasympathetic nervous system response promotes homeostasis to maintain balance and restore the body to a state where the body can repair and relax. To mindfully activate the parasympathetic nervous system one can engage in relaxing activities such as yoga, meditation, or massage. We also enter rest and digest mode when we are engaged in activities that stimulate our minds and make us feel joy.

When our body is in balance and we have the ability to think clearly and presently, we can find personal growth and enjoy a state of well-being. Participation in activities that support this type of physical, psychological, and emotional balance has been studied by psychologists who explore the school of Positive Psychology.

Many of these psychologists, such as Martin Seligman and Mihaly Csikszentmihalyi, have labeled this immersive state of optimal thoughtfulness and responsiveness as "flow." Studies have found that when people consistently engage in activities that challenge them to grow and create personally meaningful moments; they experience flow and report having an increased sense of wellbeing.

Think back to childhood, where time seemed to move slowly through the scope of your perception. Time does not speed up the older that we become; it is our perception of and interaction with time that changes. As a child, one experiences life in the present moment, forcing the brain to forge new neural pathways as it processes experiences and events in real time.

As we age, we tend to repeat the same routines on a daily basis and live in a past or future mindset. This is like holding the fast forward button down on the remote control of our cognitive functioning. We are not challenging our minds to process new information or build new thought patterns so we are passively living in the shell of our old experiences and patterns. By passively living outside of the moment, we cannot experience flow and the state of optimal wellbeing that we desire.

Finding one's flow involves a number of factors. Some questions to ask yourself when deciding whether or not you believe a certain activity promotes your wellbeing:

- Does this activity engage me in a way that brings me into the present moment, allowing me to exist outside of the linear concept of time?
- Am I utilizing a certain set of skills that I possess while being challenged in a way that prompts my skill set to evolve?
- Does this activity bring me joy and contentment?
- Do I find the action of this activity personally meaningful for its own sake?
- Am I so engaged in what I am doing that all distractions fade away?
- While engaged in this activity do I feel unselfconscious, alert, and in control?

Flow is a subjective experience and it is important to know that what creates flow for one person may not create flow for another. Some may find flow painting a picture, planting a garden, going on a run, playing a game, writing a novel, or solving a puzzle. Others may find flow through creating a charitable organization, dedicating time to their community, or designing a new video game. It is important to find your own personal flow and consistently participate in the experience of whatever activities promote this state of wellbeing.

When you choose to let go of the past and live without expectations for the future, you begin to practice non-attachment. It is only by living without attachment to the person we were yesterday or the idea of who we will become tomorrow, that we can truly allow ourselves the gift of being alive in the present moment.

When you engage in your *now*, you support your body's natural ability to maintain balance and experience optimal physical health. This healthy biological environment promotes emotional and psychological wellbeing. By living in the present moment, you free your body of unnecessary stress and create space in your life to flourish with personal growth and to experience optimal wellbeing. Find your flow, engage in your *now*, and choose a life of health and happiness.

Tips to Take on Time
Meditations and Mindset

Take a Daycation

- Do you frequently find yourself absent minded halfway through the work day?
- Does daydreaming seem like the only way to make it through the time ahead of you?
- Are you spending time ruminating about a past event or feeling anxiety about possible future events?

Then you, my friend, need a DAYCATION!

Work can seem to be the moments that blur by in between the time that we allot for our own personal development and hobbies. We get a very limited amount of time to escape from work and go on adventures or experience new things. When we consistently roll through the same motions, our brain develops a habit of not paying attention to what is occurring because the experiences are the same.

As we age, we begin to feel as if time is accelerating more rapidly when, in actuality, it is our cognition that has sped up. Because we are stuck in the same experiences daily, our brain does not have to slow down to thoroughly process what is occurring; we are skipping over the part of our personal stories that we have previously seen.

One way to live fully in the moment and overcome this skipping of time: try, on a daily basis, to experience something that causes you to pause and practice being aware. If there is a park within walking distance of your office, take a walk on your lunch break and be open to your surroundings. Engage in a new and exciting hobby after work. Take the scenic route on your morning drive or change your mode of transportation entirely.

The important thing to accomplish: find the time in your day to slow the process of cognition by having a new experience.

We may not have the luxury of jetting off to a foreign or tropical land on a whim, but that does not mean that we cannot practice living in the moment by taking mini cognitive vacations daily to boost awareness and bring ourselves fully into the present moment.

Release and Relax

When we have an experience, good or bad, we use this experience as a reference point and set expectations for future experiences. This is how we learn how to avoid bad experiences and seek out good experiences. We hoard these experiences and refuse to let go of their outcomes, even when they are no longer relevant to our lives. As children we begin to identify our role in our families and our educational systems through these experiences. As adults, we interact with the world based on the identifications we made from our experiences during the developmental stages of cognition. This is how we develop our story. This is how we gain a sense of where we came from, what we had to overcome, and where we are capable of going in the future.

Try this challenge: on a piece of paper begin to write your story or a few different experiences that you have held close to you.

- Where are you from?
- What were your hobbies growing up?
- Did you have a lot of friends in school?
- Were your dreams and desires reinforced and supported by your parents and mentors?
- Were there times you did not feel good enough?

Allow yourself to write your story without thinking. Practice flowing freely through your story. Once you have finished writing, go back and read through it once and then answer these questions:

- Do I feel my story gives an honest account of my past?
- Do I feel that my story expresses who I am, in this moment, in a positive way?
- Does this story show that I am harboring negative feelings based on these past events?
- Do I think these negative feelings, if present, prevent me from being open to new positive experiences?
- Does reading my story prompt feelings of despair, anxiety, or bitterness?
- How would letting go of this story impact my life?

Take the piece of paper on which you wrote your story and rip, crumple, or shred it then throw it into the garbage. Release yourself from the limiting thoughts that are associated with your story. Allow yourself the freedom to grow beyond the stories of your past. Experiences are gifts from which we gain the fundamental knowledge that helps us to evolve and grow. When we hold onto our stories from the past we condemn ourselves to live within their associated, limiting ideas about who we are and of what we are capable. Release and relax. You are not the thoughts that occur in your mind and you are not the person you were a second ago.

Future Foresight

Because we are creatures of habit that form experiences based on the information we collect from our physical senses, the idea of the future can be overwhelming since we cannot hold, touch, taste, see, or smell "the future." When we spend time pondering our projected possibilities of the future, based on our current or past circumstances, we experience anxiety and can develop an attachment to certain expectations or emotions. The idea that we cannot predict what is going to come next in the narrative of our personal lives can create feelings of helplessness and fear. Living in the shadow of the future, marinating in emotions that stem from conjecture based on experiences that we may never have is exhausting and counterproductive to being alive in the now!

58

Rather than living as a projection in our own possible future reality, we need to occupy the moment in which we currently exist. In order to do this, we must plan for the future one step at a time and live each day with the intention to actively create a future in alignment with our authentic self. If we set expectations in our minds, we are left to anxiously anticipate whether or not that specific outcome will occur.

To practice aligning your present with your future, enabling you to better enjoy the now, develop a morning routine that sets the intention of working towards wellness and happiness:

❖ Wake up with enough time to clear your mind of worry and really establish a clear goal of what you want to receive from your day.
❖ Plan out your week ahead of time to prevent you from getting overwhelmed by spur of the moment events and unexpected circumstances.
❖ Engage in a calming and cathartic activity, such as yoga or journaling, in order to better prepare your mind to take situations as they come.
❖ Find a sense of gratitude for your present moment and make the decision to let go of what occurred the day before.

Nature Therapy

Being surrounded by a natural landscape in which you find comfort and beauty is not only grounding but it is healing. At least once a week, take the time to get outside and be open to your surroundings. Indoors, we clutter our environment with distractions that pull us out of the present moment. Nothing can anchor us better to the present than observing nature and appreciating the strong bond that we have with our beautiful world—free of distractions like television, cellphones, computers, tablets and other technologies that have a screen. We are not a reflection of the images found on these screens, we are a direct reflection of our environment and how we choose to interact with our surroundings.

Get outside and sit in silence to observe your world. Go for a hike and engage with the ground beneath your feet and the scenery all around. Go to the beach with friends and listen to the ocean. In the winter, or if you live in a metropolis where the "great outdoors" are not a weekly option, bring the outdoors inside. House plants help to filter the air inside your home and are a great reminder to "stop and smell the roses." As a human being living on this planet, you have a right to experience the inner peace and clarity that comes from interacting with nature. Make the time to exercise this right and give yourself the gift of being a part of something larger than yourself.

Find Your Flow

On a separate sheet of paper fill in the blanks:

I am at my happiest while_____ (insert activity).

When I engage in_____ (above activity) I feel
_____, _____, and
_____.

The last time I did_____ (above activity) was
_____ (date).

I do / do not (circle one) make time to engage in this activity because_____ (list reason for doing or not doing the activity).

It is / is not (circle one) important to me to make the time to engage in activities that serve my personal growth and wellbeing.

If I could make a living from performing this activity I do / do not (circle one) feel that I would be able to partake in this activity more frequently.

When I am engaged with _____ (activity) I do / do not (circle one) feel as if I am in a state of flow where I am able to experience contentment and joy.

The purpose of this exercise is to help you focus more clearly on the important role that you play in your own happiness. Of course, our daily lives are complex and we cannot always make time for hobbies, but it is important to try and find time to dedicate to your own happiness.

When we are engaged in activities that allow us to practice creative expression, to challenge ourselves, and to experience contentment, we are truly living in the present moment. Know that you deserve to make the time to do something that serves your health, happiness and personal growth. Plan a time in your week when you can let go of the to-do-lists and enjoy something you love in the now.

Affirmations for the NOW

- ❖ I choose to release the pains of the past, the worries of the future, and to live in the present moment.

- ❖ I deserve to spend time doing the things that give me joy.

- ❖ I choose to live in the *now* and take each experience as it comes to me.

- ❖ With grace and mindfulness, I accept my life in this moment with unconditional love.

- ❖ When I live in the moment, I am able to align my actions with the intentions I hold for my health and wellness.

- ❖ In the present moment, I find health, happiness and awareness.

Occupy Your Awareness

"As we grow in our consciousness, there will be more compassion and more love, and then the barriers between people, between religions, between nations will begin to fall."

-Ram Dass

Let Go of Ego

Beginning in childhood, our behaviors were reinforced by our environment, our family members, and our peers. If we stole a toy from our friend at school, we were scolded and told to share. When we received a good grade on a spelling test, we were applauded by our parents and given a reward. Our path for behavior was either road-blocked when we behaved poorly or green-lighted when we behaved in an acceptable or desirable manner.

This reinforcement, both positive and negative, created the lasting behavioral patterns that we hold today. As we discussed in earlier sections of this book, your sense of self, your current likes or aversions, your reactionary responses, and your thought patterns are largely dependent on your previous experiences and interactions with the world. This is how we build a sense of identity, how we come to understand who we are in relation to all that surrounds us.

While it is important to have a solid sense of identity, the rigidity of placing labels and associated beliefs about self-worth can be counterproductive to personal growth and maintaining a balanced wellbeing. If I asked you to think of five adjectives to describe how you view your identity, how you view yourself in relation to the world around you, you would have very specific traits in mind—both positive and negative. If your loved ones and peers were asked to describe you using five adjectives, chances are that your view of your identity and their view of who you are in this world would differ.

Inside of your mind, someone is pretending to be you; there is a façade and a persona that has been created based on your past experiences and future projections. Although we have a tendency to believe the image we hold of ourselves in our mind to be reality, it is only a belief—a mirage that we have convinced ourselves is real. This also goes to show that our sense of identity is a subjective view of perspective and not a universally agreed-upon fact.

To create a basic illustration of this concept, think back to your favorite childhood fairytale. Children's stories tend to follow a simplistic story arch with very black-and-white characterizations. There may have been a villain holding a princess hostage, a valiant knight in shining armor, an evil witch who desires beauty and youth, or a young maiden struggling to be free of a curse.

As a child you feared the witch and villain, you were told through the story that this character was "bad" and only wanted to do evil. You rooted for the success of the knight or the freedom of the princess because they were "good" and they only wanted a happily-ever-after ending. However, if each character came to life and you had the opportunity to host an interview, you would learn that the evil witch feels she was a victim and was acting out of grief or that the knight was actually a coward and was acting out of fear.

The moral of this story is that we have developed a tendency to deduce our sense of identity into these simplistic terms; in turn, our behaviors are dependent on these rigid and incomplete views of characterization.

When we begin to attach our sense of self and identity to these beliefs and labels, we limit our potential for self-discovery and personal growth. In order to live outside the limitations of a rigid sense of self and false sense of identity, we must form our own identities based on how we live authentically in the moment; we must accept that our identity can change. One moment you may be the hero, but facing a different event, you may be the villain, and in another circumstance you may play the roles of both. The key is to raise your awareness and allow yourself the introspection to recognize the façade and shed the skin of your former self.

"Abundance is a process of letting go;
that which is empty can receive."
-Bryant H. McGill

Being open to a heightened awareness about oneself is, like all aspects of finding an optimal balance of well-being, a skill that must be practiced. Personal growth, expansion of awareness, and the transformation of health and wellbeing involve consistently being mindful of what one is thinking and how one is behaving. In addition, one must dissolve the former limiting identifications of the self.

A fundamental understanding of the unity between yourself and your environment must be formulated in order to move forward. Rather than constructing your sense of self into this façade that exists inside of your mind, dependent on associated beliefs and previous experiences, you must build your identity in unity with the external environment, or the reality in which you occupy.

When one is in tune with an authentic experience, immersed within their environment and open to the connection between oneself and one's surroundings, a higher awareness can be developed that challenges formerly held identifications. You will no longer view yourself through the unchanging and narrow lens of your own previously constructed perceptions. You will be open to really explore your identity, not as a characterization of a role within some simplistic fairytale, but rather, as an invaluable piece of all that surrounds you. Let go of your ego, free yourself of the stifling internalization of your identity, and expand beyond your own limitations.

The Occupation of Observation

Have you ever heard of the expression: *place yourself in somebody else's shoes*? This simple expression can actually become a very powerful visualization exercise. By placing yourself in someone else's life and living with the challenges of their circumstances, you can begin to develop a connection to that person. The goal in this exercise is generally to evoke feelings of empathy and compassion. You recognize one or more aspects of what the other person is experiencing as your mind directly relates similar experiences from your own life, and you begin to make a personal emotional connection.

The reason that this exercise causes such a connection to be formed is because you become the observer of someone else's pain or struggle, while discovering a fundamental and universally shared emotion at the root of the experience. You are forced to step outside of your own limiting beliefs or judgments and open your mind up long enough to realize that you and this other person, whether they may be a stranger or friend, are deeply connected in a fundamental way. You share the same emotional desire to feel love, avoid pain, and overcome whatever adversity may be present.

This type of perceptive thinking is foundational to building awareness within your own life, to expand your consciousness, and to strive toward optimal personal wellbeing. In order to truly eradicate the ego mind, or in other words further open your doors of perception, mindful observation of the self is critical. One must be in constant communication with oneself—physically, psychologically, and spiritually.

Observation of the body, of the mind, and of the spirit will build awareness of feelings, behavioral patterns, and recurring thoughts that limit the potential for wellbeing and therefore, stunt personal growth. The most essential element of practicing the life skill of observation is to recognize the difference between an observation and a thought.

While a thought could be a type of observation, our

thoughts stem from a place of belief or judgment and we tend to develop an emotional connection to our thoughts. On the other hand, observations of the self that promote growth and wellbeing stem purely from a place of authentic experience and are received without emotional attachments or judgments.

Imagine you are walking through a park. It is mid-spring and the air is perfumed with the scents of freshly cut grass and newly blossomed flowers. You stop to sit at a bench and observe that, next to your seat, the most beautiful orange Tiger Lilies are growing next to a tree. You think about how the neighbor of your childhood home had the most stunning Tiger Lilies in her large garden. You smile to yourself.

In this visualization, the observation was of the color of the flowers growing next to the tree (something you noticed within the experience of being in the park) and the thought was about your former neighbor's garden (an image that sprang to mind from a previous time in your life that evoked a particular emotional response causing you to smile).

While communicating with your body, mind and spirit, it is important to hold a space for yourself to observe without judgments or biases. While you, as the self in your life, live within a subjective reality that is unique to your senses and circumstances, you must strive to observe your reality objectively and without the attachments that bind you to counterproductive patterns.

Through yoga the practitioner learns to listen to their body and observe their breath and the physical sensations felt without judgment or attachment to those sensations (for they are only temporary and will shift as the body shifts into a different posture). Through meditation, the practitioner learns to observe their thoughts and release them without attachment (realizing that there is a separation between the person and what the person thinks about). Through the expansion of consciousness and awareness one gains insight into oneself by means of connecting to all that exists outside of one's self (realizing that the internal and the external are mirrored worlds).

If you hold onto the subjective experiences of your life and the associated beliefs or judgment—for example, holding onto the thought "I am fat," if you were previously or are currently overweight—you are preventing yourself from moving forward and changing your circumstances. You are continuously tying yourself down to the limitations of one static, emotional reaction and judgment. This type of thinking perpetuates the same type of thought patterns and behavioral patterns that have been keeping you from furthering your journey toward living a more well-balanced life and experiencing a higher state of wellbeing.

Imagine your mind is a room. In this room a stream of light is peaking through a hole in your blinds; only a tiny piece of your room is illuminated from that small stream of light. Every other inch of your room is shadowed by darkness giving you an incomplete view of your surroundings. You walk over to the window and remove the broken blind. Suddenly the room is flooded with golden sunlight, illuminating every piece of the room. You now have a complete view of our surroundings and know where you stand as a part of everything in your room. Allow this concept to apply, not only to your mind, but to your everyday interactions with your environment. Do not live with an incomplete view of your identity and of your potential to become a larger part of the whole.

> "A traveler without observation
> is a bird without wings."
> -Moslih Eddin Saadi

When one lives entirely within their incomplete perceptions, that individual becomes subject to the rules of subjective reality. By creating room for mindful observation within your life, you can recognize patterns of thought or behavior that do not serve your mission to move forward; through this recognition, you can reflect on how to better practice habits that will improve your life and serve your purpose.

This recognition and reflection then provides you with the

opportunity to take action and actually begin to walk along a balanced and prosperous path. Learning to let go of ego, live mindfully through genuine observation, and communicate with the various aspects of the self are the first steps to better occupy your awareness.

Expand to Evolve

Once you make the decision to let go of a false sense of self to begin practicing the occupation of observation, you will start to expand your perceptive reality. The same way that a tree must expand its roots in order to grow toward the sky, we must expand our awareness in order to grow toward an evolution of ourselves. The larger that we grow, the more interconnected we will become.

Once living outside the manifestations within your individualized reality you will be able to live with a heightened sense of connection to the world in which you occupy.

The Internet's intertwining connections mirror a human's mind. Through the Internet, messages are sent through cables and space, connecting individuals and organizations of people who live thousands of miles across continents and oceans. The human brain contains a large number of cable-like neurons and synapses that send electrical messages to every part of the human body, like the Internet. People utilize the Internet's vast network of connection to send and receive information from all parts of the globe throughout various moments in time.

Human consciousness is a web. While we are each one solitary synapse, or one screen connected to the ether of wireless Internet—in the universally connected brain of conscious experience—we are all a part of the larger experience of all human consciousness. Expansion of your personal awareness creates new cables for information to spread from your particular location in this web. The more aware we become as individuals, the more interconnected we become as a whole and the larger humanity's awareness can grow collectively. The broader your perceptions can grow the more connections you will be able to observe and the more you will be able to evolve on a personal level.

Being connected to this network of human perception is critical for your personal wellness. Your ability to take successful steps toward embracing a lifestyle that promotes physical wellness, psychological and emotional stability, and spiritual growth is dependent on your willingness to evolve in congruence with the interconnected web of human consciousness.

"Don't ask what the world needs.
Ask what makes you come alive, and go do it.
Because what the world needs is people who have come alive."
-Howard Thurman

You have a body that has a miraculous capacity to maintain balance and promote health. You have a mind that is capable of astounding emotional intelligence that directly impacts the state of your wellness. You live in a time in human history where every opportunity for optimal health is available. However, none of this is relevant if you do not choose to connect with the awareness to actualize your own potential to thrive.

Without awareness we live a passive and unconscious existence. In this mindset, or lack thereof, we forget to take care of our bodies, we neglect our need for continual psychological stimulation, and we surrender our capability to have meaningful and spiritual authentic life experiences. The passive life is one of physical ailment, chronic health conditions, depression, apathy, and dwindling perceptive capacity. Living unconsciously—reflexively reacting to experiences, refusing to release counterintuitive behavior and thought patterns, and stunting one's own personal growth—is like being stuck in a revolving door.

Wellness is a journey which requires constant movement, consistent action, and progressive change. We must wake up daily and make a conscious choice to work towards feeling joy, inner peace, and a hopeful positivity. When you wake up in the morning you make a decision to face your day with the intention of feeling well and finding balance, or you make the decision to be passive and out of sorts. There is no special day where clarity will strike like a lightning bolt and you will suddenly form all the habits that support a life of wellness and joy. The day that you have is today and the choice is your own.

When releasing your ego and opening yourself up to reconnect with the deeper awareness that has been buried by negative reinforcement, reactionary responses, and negligent habits, you essentially practice the idea of placing yourself in someone else's shoes; however, you are now the person with whom you need to make an empathetic connection. Viewing your subjective reality from an objective point of view can give you the perspective that you cannot see while immersed in the emotions of your own circumstances and the judgments of your own thought patterns.

You begin to realize that you are just another human being trying your best to maneuver through the world with the hope of leaving a mark and living with health and happiness along the way. Having the awareness to gain insight into your own reality sets the platform for change to become possible. In order to grow we must change and in order to change we must be mindful of our intention for the outcome of such change.

You are the pioneer of your journey. You are the warrior for your wellness. All you need to do is awaken the drive for awareness inside and make the small yet significant daily decisions that will unearth the potential for health and happiness that has always been within.

Moves to Build Momentum
Mindfulness and Modifications to Occupy Your Awareness

Simplify Your Life

Imagine that you take a drinking glass out of your cabinet and fill the glass to the brim with water. You then take a handful of pebbles and one by one, begin to drop the pebbles into the glass. As the pebbles sink to the bottom of the cup, the water will start to flow over the edges of the glass and spill out onto the floor. Despite your desire to stop the water from spilling out of the glass, you keep dropping the pebbles into the bottom until your hand is empty. You now realize how much water remains in the glass and how much water has spilled out onto the floor.

The more space in the glass that is consumed by pebbles, the less space that can be occupied by the water. You are the water. You have a desire to fill each space that you occupy with the fluid, life-force energy that exists within your body. When you are enclosed in a very small and tight space, you feel anxious and confined. And like water, when you are outside in an open field, you are free and limitless.

Now, imagine the same scene with the drinking glass except replace the word glass with the word *environment*, the word pebbles with the word *stuff*, and the word water with the word *Self*. Imagine that you are filling your environment up to the brim with stuff and that you are sacrificing space for your Self in the process. You can see that with each addition, you are losing a bit of freedom, a bit more of your own personal space to occupy, and yet you continue to fill your environment and spill your Self out over the edges. Are you willing to displace your Self in order to fill your space with more and more stuff?

Home Tour Experiment:

You decided to accept a foreign exchange student into your home. This stranger arrives from a completely different culture and looks around your home with curiosity. You give this student a tour of your house. As you walk from room to room, you begin to point out to the student the function of each room and all of the contents within the room. While explaining to the student the purpose and need for each item in your house, you find certain things more difficult to explain than others. Something that seemed a necessity when purchased has been sitting unutilized in a closet.

The room that was designed to function as a family room is dominated by an overlarge television set that prevents the family from bonding in the space. You begin to question where you fit in amongst all the stuff that seemed so essential to your life at one time. You become aware that your home has turned from a space for you to fill with your life's energy into a space that has taken your energy to fill with more and more stuff. You look at the leather couch set that was purchased on a credit card and at the surround-sound speakers you worked very hard to save up to afford.

The exchange student is looking around your home, listening to your explanations, and has a look of bewilderment on his face. You go down into your basement where your old stuff has been moved as a means for making space for your new stuff in the livable area of your home. You look around and feel a sense of bewilderment yourself. Everything that sat in the basement, collecting dust, was purchased through your hard work. You gave up a piece of your time, your energy, your Self to bring each thing in this basement into your home. You suddenly feel as much a stranger to the space you established as your home as the man standing next you from a foreign land.

When it comes to the expansion of our consciousness, to the growth of our minds and spirits, the simpler we keep our space the more available we will be to fill our lives with awareness and wellness. Practice mindfulness when you go to make a purchase. Think about what you are sacrificing to add this new pebble to your overburdened cup.

Wellness seeps deeper than maintaining your body with nutritious foods and uncluttering your mind in order to live in the now; wellness is about establishing a balance within your life that is harmonious and that encourages continual growth. Living simply opens one's life up to receive abundance while living in excess forces one into a consistent state of lack: one will consistently lack the space to house more stuff or lack the stuff to fill more space.

You are the water in the glass. You are the most profoundly essential thing in your life and you deserve to give yourself the space to live in abundance and grow beyond the limitations that you build around yourself.

Serve Your Spirit

The term *spirituality* can be polarizing. Many people associate the idea of being spiritual with the idea of belonging to a specific religious group or ideology. When it comes to classifying yourself as a spiritual or non-spiritual person, you may reflect upon the last time that you attended a religious ceremony or celebrated an associated traditional holiday.

However, spirituality and religion are not one in the same. Religious people can be non-spiritual and people who do not practice a religion can be spiritual. While some definitions may claim that spirituality pertains to things of an ecclesiastical nature, the root word of this definition is "spirit". The term spirit refers to anything that has to do with the principle of conscious life or the incorporeal piece of the human being. In this regard, identifying as a spiritual person means that one serves their consciousness and places value on the immaterial piece of their being.

Wellness includes health of the body, peace of the mind, and vitality of the spirit: a balance between each form of the human being. Only you can know how to best serve your soul and invest in the expansion of your consciousness. You have the capacity to develop a practice that reinforces your spirit and that brings vitality into your life. The primary focus of your spiritual practice should be to bring nourishment to your conscious body, feeding your awareness and expanding your perceptions. You can engage in religious practices and still have a separate spiritual practice that focuses on enriching the core of your personal life in different ways.

Art can be a spiritual practice. Through the process of creating art, one gains insight into the essence of something, someone, or some situation that can be related to the essence of one's own spirit. The creative process acts as a vehicle for the artist to transcend the limited and subjective perception of the individual reality and relate to an expanded awareness that causes self-introspection and challenges growth in a proactive and conscious manner. This process of creation is both spiritually nourishing and consciously stimulating. As a result, the individual becomes more aware of their personal connection to the world at large and the universal energy that flows through all things.

Any activity that engages you to gain insight into your connection to the collective consciousness and build lasting relationships to these insights, to enrich your own capacity for enlightenment, can be considered a spiritual practice. The key is to stay consistent and devoted.

Pick a day and time each week when you will engage in your own spiritual practice. It is important that you view this time as sacred. Make a commitment to serve your spirit during this time and try, to the best of your ability, to consistently engage in this practice. Be it meditation, prayer, art, reading, walking in nature, or practicing yoga, make the decision that you deserve to serve your spirit and nourish your life.

Observation Journal

Through yoga, the practitioner learns how to observe how their minds observe their bodies. For example, when you begin something new, you may have thoughts such as *I am not good at this activity* or *I don't know why I bother*. When you pay attention to these thoughts, you choose to exit the present moment; you choose to live inside of your mind, and as a result, you miss out on having an authentic experience.

In yoga, the practitioner learns to detach themselves from the thoughts that will undoubtedly arise in one's mind by paying close attention to how one is breathing and how one's body is moving through the flow of postures. Applying this idea of *observing the observer* to your daily life will enable you to live fully within the moment and have more impactful life experiences.

Learning to dissociate your identity from the thoughts that you have about yourself is not an easy task. We have been brought up to identify the thoughts in our head as the voice of our life narrative. When we attach to these thoughts and believe them to be the voice of who we are as people, our entire identity is formulated around the beliefs we have held about ourselves.

You need to make an active and conscious effort to recognize your thoughts as words in your head and not allow them to define who you are as a being. Paying attention to these thoughts limits the interaction you have with the moment at hand and therefore, limits how you will develop and grow from the experience. To practice living as an observer in your own life, start an Observation Journal.

How to Utilize an Observation Journal:

❖ Practice writing in a free form and write whatever thoughts come to your mind. Seeing these thoughts on paper will help you gain perspective on what value you place on them and the role that they play in your life.

76

❖ Take the journal with you when you leave the house. When you have a moment of free time, rather than playing a game on your phone or chatting with a coworker, write down everything you can observe about your surroundings. What smells surround you? Does the lighting make you feel comfortable? What are the other people in your surroundings doing? Do you feel hungry? What colors are painted on the walls? Any detail that allows you to observe the moment, write it down.

❖ Pick an item in your environment and write down how you would describe the item to a person who cannot experience it firsthand. Be very descriptive.

❖ Remember a happy memory you have from your childhood and write down every detail that you can remember. Observe how this memory makes you feel in the present moment; how your body reacts physically and what thoughts are associated with the memory.

These are just a few examples of how to use an Observation Journal as a tool to build awareness and detach from limiting beliefs. Feel free to use this journal in the ways that best suit your needs. Again, like many aspects of wellness discussed in this book, **consistency is the key.** Wellness is a continual journey that requires your consistent, active participation.

Practice Kindness

Growing up, you may have been told to treat others how you would like to be treated. This is a fantastic concept that focuses on building a community where people feel empathy and place themselves in the shoes of other people. When it comes to expanding your awareness to better your own health, and the health of your community, it should also be said to treat **yourself** how you would like to be treated. By focusing on being kind to others we can lose touch with how to be kind to ourselves. Self-love and self-care are not practices that should be viewed as selfish.

By definition, in order to be considered selfish one must be acting to solely serve a personal purpose with a disregard for others. When we practice self-love and self-care we are serving ourselves in order to better serve others. It is important to realize that by being the most healthful and happy version of yourself, you will be able to better serve the health and happiness of every other person in your life.

Kindness Exercise:

On sticky notes or a piece of paper to hang on your wall, write down 5 things that you love about yourself:

1._____
2._____
3._____
4._____
5._____

Next, write down 5 things that other people love about you:

1._____
2._____
3._____ _____
4._____
5._____

Lastly, write down a negative thought that you have held about yourself and then write why you deserve to let go of that thought:

I have always thought that I _____
_____ but I choose to release this false belief about myself because I am deserving of love and
_____.

Each day try and remind yourself why you are deserving of self-love and why you deserve to work towards feeling healthy and happy. Ultimately, you are the one person who will set the standard for how you want to be treated and how you will be able to treat others.

One cannot learn to swim by refusing to let go of the side of the pool. You cannot work towards building awareness, expanding consciousness, and living in wellness if you are holding onto false and negative beliefs about yourself that will limit your potential for growth.

Be Proactive, Not Reactive

Think about the last time you procrastinated and wound up in a situation that could have been prevented if you choose to take action instead of waiting to be forced into action. When we wait to have a situation force our hand into motion, we tend to have less options to solve the situation and are stressed by the necessity of a speedy solution. When we choose procrastination, we fall into a pattern of reacting to events at the last minute. This leads us to feel overwhelmed and stressed, limiting our foresight to plan ahead for the next series of events. Once this cycle begins, it becomes increasingly difficult to end. We are constantly struggling to muster the energy to solve the immediate problem when the next one is already on our heels.

Through mindfulness, one can combat the effects that stress plays on health by proactively preventing stressful situations or by handling stressors when they do occur. By choosing to handle situations with mindfulness and clarity, you can dramatically improve your health and wellbeing. Practicing mindfulness outside of stressful situations will better prepare your mind and body to better handle immediate stressors when they arise. You have the capability to directly impact the biological chemistry of your body. You may not be able to choose what circumstances you will face but you are in control of how you handle the circumstances and how you allow them to affect your health.

Affirmations for Awareness

- ❖ I choose to live in awareness: to be mindful and present in each moment.

- ❖ Through meditation, I find clarity and peace of mind.

- ❖ I choose to be kind to myself and practice self-care.

- ❖ I recognize negative thoughts that limit my growth but choose to release these thoughts from my mind.

- ❖ I embrace the abundance which the Universe provides to me.

- ❖ With clarity and patience I observe myself in the moment and embrace living in the now.

- ❖ My mind is open and available to expand and grow.

Occupy Your Life

Progress is The Process

Living in harmony with your health involves discovering a balance on all levels of your personal wellness. On a physical level, you must feed your body to nourish your organs, to cleanse your tissues, and animate your limbs with life. To unclutter your mind and liberate your life from negative thought patterns, you must live with mindfulness in the now. Inner peace can only come from expanding your mind and evolving your awareness. To the logical mind, this may seem to be overwhelming. But because all of these moving parts are connected, balance comes more rapidly with each small turn of one piece.

Feeling better in your body will ultimately lead you to live more authentically in the moment and have the awareness to observe genuine life experiences that both perpetuate personal growth and bring purpose and joy into your life. The simple exercises, affirmations, and mediations provided in the previous pages are powerful tools to begin redirecting the intentions for health in your life. The key is to be consistent in your actions and remember your reasoning; remind yourself daily how feeling well and finding joy from within will dramatically improve your life. You must advocate for your health and you must put in whatever it is that you wish to get out.

You deserve to wake up and feel well. Your body was designed to flourish and you are capable of aiding in your own healing. You are a conscious being living in this world, in the now. You are alive with an ever-expanding consciousness that connects you to the world. There is no thing, nor is there any person, that can deny you the right to wake up and choose wellness—except for yourself.

You deserve to live free from ailment, from negativity, and from unhappiness. Begin your path by setting the intention to start implementing new patterns for wellness in your life.

In yoga, the practitioner will perform the same stretches consistently and while holding the posture, the practitioner will lengthen the spine on an inhale and deepen the posture on an exhale. This wave-like movement is controlled by taking very conscious and deliberate breaths. Small incremental motions will, over time, allow the practitioner to exceed personal boundaries and move on to master more intricate stretches and postures.

The progress is truly realized after the practitioner has continued to practice the same postures consistently. Patience, awareness, self-love, acceptance, and discipline: these are all traits that the practitioner must possess to propel forward. There is mindfulness within every little movement taken towards deepening one's practice; it is all part of the process and it is the only way to gain any progress.

No one can dictate the idea of what wellness means to you personally or how you need to go about working towards becoming well. You must listen to your body, mind and spirit in order to set the intention for yourself and begin to take the action steps that will lead you down your path to freedom. The more individuals who begin to embark down their path to balance and vitality, the more our global community will grow and thrive. As in your own body, the elements for wellness are foundational and interconnected on a global scale.

"Changes and progress rarely are gifts from above.
They come out of struggles from below."
-Noam Chomsky

Through my personal journey for health, I acquired a lot of knowledge and, after I began to feel well enough, I began helping others discover their drive for discovering balance, health and happiness. When you are feeling great inside of your body, clear within your mind, and enlightened in spirit, it is impossible not to form a strong desire to share all that you can with others. You begin to radiate health and your positive energy becomes magnetic. You will become a beacon—a light for others who may be lost on their path.

Revolutionizing your personal wellness is the best way to begin a global revolution for change. Like wildfire, the positive energy of people who feel well inside of their bodies and joy within their lives spreads from person to person and place to place. Through technology, our world is becoming smaller, but our problems are becoming larger. We have had the ultimate tool for constructing a better world within us all along—our innate and miraculous desire to thrive. Each person who chooses to heed this call on a daily basis, though it may seem small, begins to slowly aid in the healing of our global body.

Once you begin to eat well, you may feel a desire to start a community garden or to advocate for a healthier public school lunch program in your county. When you eat well and feel well, you will have the ability to focus on building up the world around you and expanding the limitations of your old reality. Maybe this will drive you to run a local art exhibition or to host a benefit show where local businesses will get to participate. With the awareness you build through mindful living, you will outgrow the current circumstances that have left you feeling stuck and, instead, find a desire to travel the world or open your doors of perception, thus leaving positive vibrations in your wake.

We deserve to wake up and feel well. Our global body was designed to flourish and we are capable of aiding in our own healing. We are conscious beings living in this world, in the now. We are alive with an ever-expanding consciousness that connects us to our world. There is no person who can deny us the right to wake up and choose wellness, except for ourselves. We deserve to live free from ailment, from negativity, and from unhappiness. We must begin our path by setting the intention to start implementing new patterns for wellness in our lives.

Warrior Wellness by Kimberly Ann

Biography

After graduating from Hofstra University with a Bachelor of Arts degree in Creative Writing and a minor in Psychology, I attended the Institute for Integrative Nutrition™. During my training, I studied over 100 dietary theories, practical lifestyle management techniques, and innovative coaching methods with some of the world's top health and wellness experts. My teachers included: Dr. Andrew Weil, Director of the Arizona Center for Integrative Medicine; Dr. Deepak Chopra, leader in the field of mind-body medicine; Dr. David Katz, Director of Yale University's Prevention Research Center; Dr. Walter Willett, Chair of Nutrition at Harvard University; Geneen Roth, bestselling author and expert on emotional eating; and many other leading researchers and nutrition authorities.

My education has equipped me with extensive knowledge in holistic nutrition, health coaching, and preventive health. Drawing on these skills and my knowledge of different dietary theories, I work with clients to help them make lifestyle changes that produce real and lasting results. Upon graduation, I became a board certified Holistic Health Practitioner with the American Association of Drugless Practitioners and furthered my education by studying the practice of yoga as a Yoga Alliance registered yoga teacher.

Following my passion to better serve all of my clients and expand the Warrior Wellness tribe, I continue to study various aspects of wellness and acquire a broader range of tools. *Occupy Your Body* has been my first book released as a published author but it will not be my last.

Mission

At the start of 2015, I established Warrior Wellness by Kimberly Ann. Not only do I have a drive to help my peers and clients embark on a journey for personal wellness, I have a vision of building a thriving tribe and community of empowered, healthy and happy individuals who are dedicated to evolving personally and revolutionizing the health of the world.

Through Warrior Wellness, it is my mission to help establish a more healthful global community by helping each individual client align their lifestyle with their authentic drive for total wellness of the body, mind and spirit. Through the implementation of real-world tools, such as yoga, mindful eating, and meditation, I help my clients build permanent and healthful lifestyle habits that will help prevent chronic health conditions, promote physical wellbeing, and improve overall quality of life.

It is my intention through Warrior Wellness by Kimberly Ann, to teach you time effective and practical tools that can be practiced on a daily basis to improve the quality of life for yourself, your family, and your community. I strongly believe that each individual has the capacity to better their life and the responsibility to better the health of the budding global tribe of humanity. Individually, we can grow together, and together we can impact the world.

Services
Health Coaching:

- Personalized Wellness Programs
- Group Wellness Programs
- Corporate Wellness Programs
- Weight Management
- Nutritional Cleansing Programs

Yoga:

- Personalized Asana Practice
- Group Asana Programs
- Corporate Yoga

Meditation and Spirituality:

- Private or Group Meditation Seminars
- Spiritual Exploration
- Guided Meditations

Speaker and Author:

- Holistic Living Blog
- Seminars and Lectures on Various Health Related Topics
- Online Health Workshops and Wellness Seminars

For details on all the services and programs offered by Warrior Wellness please visit my website and blog at www.unearthyourwarrior.com. Feel free to contact me via E-mail at wellnesswithkimberly@gmail.com and connect with me on Facebook, Twitter, and other social media sources.

Become a Warrior for Your Wellness

Why Warrior Wellness?

Well, that is a good question.

What if I asked you to envision yourself as a warrior?

What comes to mind?

My guess is that you imagine yourself as a large and powerful person ornate with armor, weapons, and a fierce countenance. This, in terms of my intentions through Warrior Wellness, is not entirely accurate. A true wellness warrior does not utilize a weapon-laden defense to take back their health, but rather seeks resolution and evolution through an internal authentic offense.

We cannot change our health by taking on the established systems and attempting to make changes in our external world. Instead, we need to become warriors and advocates for changing ourselves from within in order to change the world. In order to achieve true wellness, the fiercest warrior uses the ultimate tools of discipline, inner peace, acceptance of the Self and of circumstances, and compassionate understanding. After all, what good is a sword with armor without the knowledge and skills necessary to wield it? Rather than conquering through brute force, one must seek authentic health through a meditative understanding of the self.

"As human beings, our greatness lies not so much in being able to remake
the world—that is the myth of the atomic age—
as in being able to remake ourselves."
-Ghandi

What if I asked you to envision your inner wellness warrior again?

87

Does the vision change?

Do you see yourself sitting in quiet reflection in a serene garden, or doing yoga by a lake?

There is a warrior of wellness inside of you, formed from your natural and organic drive to wake up feeling energized, fit, and happy. Every day you can make the choice to either nurture or ignore this warrior drive.

Will you make the choice to be authentic to yourself, to your truth, to live mindfully in the moment and fully occupy this body you have been given in the now?

Take action today. Join the Warrior Wellness tribe and unearth your warrior within.

Namasté

I honor the place in you in which the entire Universe dwells
The place of Love, of Truth, of Light & of Peace
When you are in that place in you and I am in that place in me
We Are One.

Gratitude is the Attitude

As I do at the end of each yoga class that I teach, I am sharing with you my deepest gratitude. Thank you for allowing me to participate in your growth, in your light, and in your life. It is my sincerest hope that you utilize all the information that I have shared in this book and begin embarking on your journey to wellness, mindful living, and authentic happiness.

As you grow, I grow, and together we evolve as a united and harmonious humanity. I am forever grateful for this opportunity I have been given to help support you, as a partner and teacher, on your continual journey to balanced and authentic living.

Thank you.

Occupy Your Body.
Occupy Your NOW.
Occupy Your Awareness.
You are Deserving.
You are Complete.
You are in Balance.

We are Whole.
We Are The 100%.

Flow of References

1. Lurz, Robert. Animal Minds. *Internet Encyclopedia of Philosophy*. ISSN 2161-0002. Web. 7/22/2015

2. Ward BW, Schiller JS, Goodman RA.. Multiple Chronic Conditions Among US Adults: A 2012 update. *Center for Disease Control and Prevention*. Web. 7/22/2015

3. The Editors of Encyclopedia Britannica. Sisyphus: Greek Mythology. *The Encyclopedia Britannica*. Web. 7/30/2015

4. Eveleth, Rose. There are 37.2 Trillion Cells in Your Body. *Smithsonian Smart News*. 10/24/2013. Web. 8/6/2015

5. IPAC. What Are Stars Made of? *Cool Cosmos*. Web. 8/6/2015 http://coolcosmos.ipac.caltech.edu/ask/205-What-are-stars-made-of-

6. Martin Ben, Psy.D. In-Depth: Cognitive Behavioral Therapy. *PsychCentral*. Web. 8/6/2015

7. Collective Unconscious: Psychology. *The Encyclopedia Britannica*. The Encyclopedia Britannica, Inc. Web. 8/12/2015

8. Hadhazy, Adam. Think Twice: How the Gut's "Second Brain" Influences Mood and Wellbeing. *Scientific American*. Division of Nature America, Inc. 2/12/2010. Web. 8/20/2015

9. Gina Shaw. Reviewed by Brunilda Nazario, MD. Water and Your Diet: Staying Slim and Regular with H2O. *WebMD*. WebMD, LLC 07/07/2009. Web. 8/24/2015.

10. Madhav Goyal, MD, MPH[1]; Sonal Singh, MD, MPH[1]; Erica M. S. Sibinga, MD, MHS[2]; et al. Meditation Programs for Psychological Stress and Well-being. *JAMA Network*. JAMA Internal Medicine, 03/2014. Web. 8/24/2015.

11. Prescott Gregg, M.S. Carl Jung- The Man Who Coined The Word "Synchronicity". *IN5D*. Esoteric, Metaphysical, and Spiritual Database, 01/19/2015. Web. 9/2/2015

12. Physics and Consciousness: Quantum Interconnectedness. *StarStuffs*. Nature of Mind, Body, and Spirit, 10/12/2014. Web. 9/2/2015.

13. Mercola Joseph, MD. Falling for This Myth Could Give You Cancer. *Mercola.com*. 04/11/2012. Web. 9/2/2015.

14. Institute for Stem Cell Biology and Regenerative Medicine. *Stanford Medicine*. Research. Web. 9/21/2015.

15. Positive Psychology. *The Positive Psychology People*. Research. Web. 9/22/2015.

16. PBS. Flow. *This Emotional Life*. Vulcan Productions, 2011. Web. 9/22/2015

www.ingramcontent.com/pod-product-compliance
Lightning Source LLC
Chambersburg PA
CBHW032117280326

41933CB00009B/885